.

Food is Foundational

A Workbook to Identify your Nutritional Needs

Tammy Westney, MS, CPT

For my mother Judy and grandmother Rita

Introduction

Introduction

I grew up in the 1960s and 1970s, at a time when processed foods were just beginning to catch on. As a young child I remember my grandmother cooking soups for hours with bones left over from a previous meal. We waited with barely contained anticipation for the first summer tomatoes, corn, and watermelons. Back then our available food was dependent on the season. I still remember how wonderful they tasted.

I also remember the introduction of TV dinners, Hamburger Helper, and Captain Crunch. It was our fault, my brother and I, we saw it on TV and begged for it. Then McDonalds came to a town not far from our home and Burger King was not far behind. Though these were all rare and special treats for us. It was a changing foodscape, and not for the better.

We were fortunate in our multigenerational house. My grandmother was far ahead of her time. She would not have soda in our house, anything with dyes were also prohibited. Had she learned about preservatives, we probably wouldn't have had the Hamburger Helper either.

Sadly, processed foods have become so ingrained in the way we eat, that this way of eating is known as the Standard American Diet (SAD). This type of diet is notoriously low in nutrient density and has been implicated in the development of chronic inflammatory diseases and chronic illnesses such as heart disease and arthritis, stroke, cancer, diabetes, and obesity. The most problematic foods in this kind of diet are processed foods, foods high in sugar, and foods high in saturated fat.

It should come as no surprise that food can also have as direct an effect on our mental health as it does on our physical health. Consider the fact that the blocked veins struggling to bring blood to your heart, are struggling to bring blood to your brain as well. Long-term this contributes to overall cognitive decline, dementia, and Alzheimer's disease. Changes in your brain structure can be seen ten years before any symptoms appear.

Developing a new pattern of healthy eating requires a shift in the way we look at food. Food is information. Your cells don't know what to do with processed food. But give your body an apple or carrot and your body knows exactly what to do with that fuel.

The next time you're in the supermarket try to reframe your idea of fast food. Consider the produce aisle as your new drive-through. Tomatoes, rich in lycopene, can be the base of many good meals. Shredded zucchini makes a terrific substitute for low-nutrient pasta. Organic fruit is the ultimate fast-food, just rinse and eat!

When my grandmother was a child people ate like traditional cultures eat today. Local, whole foods are picked fresh or preserved through fermentation or drying methods. Traditional cultures generally remain free of chronic disease.

Food is Foundational. We are what we eat right down to our cells and without the proper fuel the cardiovascular system, digestive system and our metabolic pathways will all be seriously affected.

Part One

Chapter One

Basic Nutritional Needs, Macronutrients

Not all calories are equal. Fats are the most calorically dense food, they slow down the digestive process keeping you full longer. Proteins are not as calorically dense as fats. They provide the amino acids which are the building blocks of our cells. Complex carbohydrates have the same caloric density as protein, but they break down into glucose which rapidly fuels our cells.

The amino acids that make up protein are used by our cells for reproduce and repair. There are 20 amino acids, nine of which are essential amino acids. A complete protein is comprised of the nine essential amino acids that the body cannot make on its own. Animal protein sources are complete proteins this includes meat, cheese, eggs, and sea food.

Amino acids are found in other foods and they can be combined to make a meal that includes all the essential amino acids. Think of the cultures using variations of beans and rice. You can find lentils and rice, soy beans and rice, black or white beans, chick or black eyed peas. Other plant sources include quinoa, nuts, and seeds. These can also be combined with grains to create complete proteins.

Carbohydrates have gotten a lot of bad press in recent years. However, they are an important part of a healthy diet. It's important to remember that you need complex carbohydrates, they break down slowly, unlike simple or refined carbohydrates, which break down quickly and can leave you hungry and experiencing a sugar crash.

Include complex carbohydrates in your diet, grains like barley, oats and brown rice. Beans and legumes, which are also form of protein and are filled with fiber.

Vegetables like leafy greens, root vegetables, and fruits all add phytonutrients and antioxidants to your diet.

If you add some fat like butter or olive oil and some protein, it will slow down the digestion even more. Leaving you with sustained energy and no hunger pains!

Fat is vital to every cell in our bodies, it makes up the phospholipid bilayer which surrounds and protects cells. Fat soluble vitamins need fat in order to be absorbed.

Some healthy sources of fat include coconut oil which is anti-viral, anti-bacterial and anti-fungal. It is made of medium chain fatty acids, which can be used quickly for energy, and are rarely stored as fat. There are two varieties, virgin has the flavor of a coconut, and filtered is neutral-tasting

Organic Butter has short, and medium chain, saturated, monounsaturated and polyunsaturated fatty acids. It contains fat-soluble vitamins A, D and E. Clarified butter is also known as ghee, which is well-tolerated because the milk solids are removed. Ghee does not have to be refrigerated because it has so many antioxidants and no milk solids.

Olive oil is high in monounsaturated fat. MUFAs, can help lower your cholesterol. According to the New England Journal of Medicine consuming four tablespoons daily can lower the risk of having a heart attack, suffering a stroke or dying of heart disease. Olive oil is full of polyphenols, an antioxidant that can help protect your cells from damage. (27)

Many foods fit into more than one category, like beans which are both a carbohydrate and protein. These delicious whole foods are good sources of both healthy fats and proteins, nuts, cheese, seeds, fish and eggs.

Macronutrient Requirements

The debate over macronutrient requirements rages on in the form of competing diet trends. High protein, low carbohydrate and high fat diets have all been in the news. It can all be confusing to someone who would just like a healthy diet.

When considering your caloric needs you need to consider your level of activity. An average person leading a sedentary life would only need about 1,800 calories a day to maintain their current weight. If that same person led an active life they would need 2,300 calories, and if they were very active they would need 2,600.

Protein and carbohydrates each have 4 calories per gram and fat has 9 calories. To calculate your needs multiply your target by the percentage you'd like to consume 2,000 x.51=1,020. Divide 1,020 by the macronutrient 1,020 / .04 = 255.

The USDA has an interactive calculator to help you estimate your caloric, macronutrient, vitamin and mineral needs. Go to the USDA website and use the interactive DRI for healthcare professionals. There you can list your gender, age, height and weight and it will calculate your nutritional needs.

If you are interested in guidelines, the USDA basic requirements for a person consuming 2,000 calories a day are:

Carbohydrates:	Protein:	Fat:
51% of your diet or 255 grams	18% or 90 grams	33% or 73 grams

If you wanted to try a high protein diet the 2,000 calories a day are:

Carbohydrates:	Protein:	Fat:
10% of your diet or 200 grams	30% or 150 grams	30% or 67 grams

If you wanted to try a high fat or ketogenic diet the 2,000 calories a day are:

Carbohydrates:	Protein:	Fat:
5% of your diet or 10 grams	25% or 50 grams	70% or 140 grams

Speak with your doctor before making radical changes to your diet. Some of these diets could be harmful depending on your health status. For instance high protein diets would not be recommended to anyone with kidney or liver concerns.

Here's a quiz to see if you are deficient in macronutrients. Do you have or experience:

1. __ Dry skin
2. __ Reduced visual acuity
3. __ Rough bumpy skin on arms
4. __ Cracked heels
5. __ Eczema
6. __ Thick calluses
7. __ Dandruff
8. __ Thin, weak, cracked fingernails
9. __ Memory problems
10. __ Thin sparse hair
11. __ Hair is dull, dry, or brittle
12. __ Band or patches of hair lighter in color
13. __ Hair pulls out easily with no pain
14. __ Muscle wasting or shrinking
15. __ Decreased grip strength
16. __ Brown patches on face
17. __ Red gums
18. __ Ridged, flattened, or spooned shaped fingernails

Numbers 1-9 indicate low essential fatty acids. If you checked off more than 4 of these you may be deficient in essential fatty acids.

Numbers 10-18 indicate low protein. If you checked off more than 4 you may be protein deficient.

Basic Nutritional Needs, Micronutrients

Vitamin and mineral deficiencies can lead to serious problems. Blood testing can be performed to confirm suspected deficiencies, however many people live with a series of increasingly problematic symptoms before seeking treatment.

We need Vitamin A Retinol, Vitamin A Carotenoids, Vitamin B1 Thiamin, Vitamin B2 Riboflavin, Vitamin B3 Niacin, Vitamin B5 Pantothenic Acid, Vitamin B6 Pyridoxine, Vitamin B9 Folic Acid, Vitamin B12 Cobalamin, Vitamin C Ascorbic Acid, Vitamin D Cholecalciferol, Vitamin E Tocopherol, and Vitamin K.

The minerals we need include Calcium, Copper, Chromium, Iodine, Iron, Magnesium, Manganese, Phosphorus, Potassium, Selenium, Sodium, and Zinc.

These are some of my favorite Super foods:

Broccoli is high in Vitamins C and K, as well as Manganese.

Beets are high in Folate, Vitamin C, Potassium, and Manganese.

Sweet Potato: are high in Vitamins A, C, B6, Potassium, and Copper.

Dark Leafy Greens like kale or spinach are high in Vitamins A, B1, B6, B9, C, and K.

Lentils are high in Vitamins B1, B6, B9, Phosphorus, Potassium, and Zinc.

Peppers are also high in both Vitamins C, K, B6, and A.

Tuna is high in Vitamin A, Snapper in B12, Trout and Salmon are high in Vitamin D.

Nuts like Almonds and Pecans are high in B1 and A Vitamins.

Sea vegetables like wakame also high in many of the same vitamins as leafy greens and have the added benefit of iodine, and potassium.

Here's a quiz to see if you have any vitamin or mineral deficiencies.

Do you have or experience:

1. __ Vision dysfunctions, Night blindness, Dry skin and eyes
2. __ Insomnia, Headache, Memory loss, Noise sensitivity
3. __ Hair loss, Dermatitis, Chapped lips, Cracks in corners of mouth
4. __ Red sore tongue, Fatigue, Weakness
5. __ Restless, Poor healing, Burning feet and hands
6. __ Fatigue, Dark patches on face
7. __ Anemia, Red, slick tongue, Loss of balance
8. __ Bleeding gums, Poor healing, Bruising
9. __ Profuse sweating, Low Calcium, Scaly lips
10. __ Dry hair, Age spots, Impaired reflexes
11. __ Prolonged blood clotting times, Hemorrhaging
12. __ Decreased bone density, Osteoporosis, Tooth decay
13. __ Intolerance to cold, Low body temperature, Weight gain
14. __ Anemia, Fatigue, Spoon nails
15. __ Muscle cramps, Hypertension, Sugar cravings,
16. __ Excessive thirst, Muscle pain, irregular heartbeat.
17. __ Low blood pressure, Abdominal bloating , Dizziness, Headache
18. __ White spots on nails, Loss of taste, increased susceptibility to infection

If you any of these symptoms on a regular basis, see a doctor. These can be sign of serious problems that should be treated by a professional.

Answer Key:

1. Vitamin A Retinol
2. Vitamin B1 Thiamin
3. Vitamin B2 Riboflavin
4. Vitamin B3 Niacin
5. Vitamin B6 Pyridoxine
6. Vitamin B9 Folic Acid
7. Vitamin B12 Cobalamin
8. Vitamin C Ascorbic Acid
9. Vitamin D Cholecalciferol
10. Vitamin E Tocopherol
11. Vitamin K
12. Calcium
13. Iodine
14. Iron
15. Magnesium
16. Potassium.
17. Sodium
18. Zinc

Chapter Two

Digestion

The human body has evolved into a finely tuned organism. Take for instance the digestive system, when it is working properly it can take a meal and break the carbohydrates down into glucose, break protein into amino acids and take fat and break it into fatty acids.

Digestion begins in your mouth, where you mechanically breakdown food by chewing it. There is also a secretion in your saliva called salivary amylase, which begins to breakdown carbohydrates before they even reach your stomach.

The stomach is where food is chemically broken down into chime, a liquid mix of food and gastric juices. Having the proper level of hydrochloric acid (HCl) is important for killing pathogens, and to break down the nutrients in your food.

The small intestine functions as the gatekeeper. When it is working properly it absorbs nutrients from the chime as it passes. It also blocks the absorption of non-foods like chemicals and bacteria, as well as food that has not been adequately broken down. This process takes place in the villi and microvilli which line the small intestines. Each of the three parts of the small intestine, the duodenum, jejunum, and the ilium absorbs different nutrients.

The Colon is home to the microbiome. A healthy microbiome acts to break down fibrous food, produce vitamins, increase the absorption of minerals balance your intestinal pH, and produce short-chain fatty acids. The food you eat can help or hurt your microbes leading to either a healthy microbiome or one that is compromised by dysbiosis, which is an imbalance flora of the microbiome.

Common Digestive Disorders

Gastroesophageal Reflux Disease (GERD)

GERD is the result of the damage to the lower esophageal sphincter. This sphincter opens to allow food into the stomach. When it doesn't properly close, acid from the stomach can escape into the esophagus causing a burning sensation.

Causes for GERD include:

Being overweight

Sitting with a slumped posture

Having food sensitivities

Eating too close to bedtime

In the past people were told to change their eating habits in order to avoid the symptoms of GERD. However with the advent of proton-pump inhibitors (PPIs) that is no longer necessary. These drugs act to decrease the production of stomach acid.

However, the problem with PPIs is that you need to have stomach acid. It cleans your food, keeps you from developing dysbiosis and it is necessary to break down your food to get the nutrients you need.

Chronic diseases are also linked to use of non-steroidal anti-inflammatory drugs. These include an increased possibility of developing upper and lower gastrointestinal bleeding, and increased cardiovascular risks. The damage to the gastrointestinal tract can be quite severe. The types of damage seen include perforation, obstruction, as well as clinically significant anemia.

If you want to try natural remedies give marshmallow root and aloe juice a try, as these are stomach soothing. Another option is sodium or potassium bicarbonate mixed in water. These can provide relief by raising the stomach's ph.

The best treatment for GERD is to maintain your ideal weight, be aware of your posture, pay attention to what you eat, avoid foods that upset your stomach, and don't eat close to bedtime.

Increased Intestinal Permeability

Leaky Gut is seen when the endothelial cells lining the digestive tract are damaged. Food cannot be properly digested, which leads to partially digested food particles in the bloodstream.

Once these food particles enter the blood stream the immune system targets these "foreign" objects. It creates antibodies, which lead to the development of reactions to common foods.

Causes:

Chronic stress

Dysbiosis

Exposure to toxins

Heavy alcohol consumption

Poor food choices

Nonsteroidal drugs

Food sensitivities

Elimination diets can be helpful in treating this disorder. It will take at least 3 months for the intestines to heal. See the section on Bone broth.

Candida

Candida is a yeast-like fungus, which is commonly present in your intestines. Its growth is usually limited by your immune system and by your micro flora, the "good" microbes lining in your digestive tract.

Candida can become problematic when the immune system is weakened, resulting in intestinal candidiasis. This overgrowth can become systemic leading to thrush in the mouth and throat, vaginal infections, and skin eruptions.

Causes:

Repeated use of antibiotics, oral contraceptives, and/or steroids like prednisone

Diet high in sweets

Alcohol

Chronic stress

Diabetes

Weakened immune system

Making some changes to your diet can make a big difference in your recovery from this imbalance. Foods that are high in carbohydrates (sugar) will need to be eliminated.

Peanuts and pistachios should also be avoided. They tend to be high in mold, which can worsen Candida.

Mushrooms which are also in the fungus family should be avoided.

Fermented foods such as vinegar and aged cheeses can feed the Candida and should be avoided.

These foods should be avoided for at least 2-4 weeks. If after reintroducing these foods symptoms reoccur, remove them from the diet for 2-3 months.

Diverticulitis

Diverticulitis is the development of pockets, usually within the colon, which collect waste particles. Most people remain symptom free. However, when the pockets become inflamed, symptoms can include cramping, diarrhea, fever, and even blood in the stool. This can be extremely serious. Seek medical treatment if you have or suspect you have diverticulitis.

Treatment is targeted to first treat the infection. At this time a low fiber diet is recommended. During the second stage of treatment a high fiber diet can be reintroduced. A diet high in fiber is important for two reasons: it improves stool motility, and it feeds the microflora within the colon.

Use of products such as Beano, which provides enzymes to digest food that can cause gas, also reduces the amount fiber that the colon needs to stay healthy.

Some natural remedies include:

Mucilaginous herbs such as slippery elm, which improves stool motility and enhances colon flora.

Spasmolytics like cramp bark, wild yam, and chamomile decrease pain associated with spasms.

Herbs that increase the strength of the colon wall include grape seed extract, and hawthorn.

Immune enhancing herbs, such as echinacea and andrographis can work to control infection.

Anti-inflammatory herbs, like meadowsweet and chamomile work directly on the gastrointestinal tract.

Gastrointestinal antiseptics will encourage the growth of normal flora.

Fatty Liver Disease

Fatty liver disease is a condition that occurs when spaces in the liver where blood would normally flow instead fill up with fat. These fat pockets reduce the flow of nutrients to the liver cell. Inflammation develops and the liver cells can even rupture.

Fatty liver can develop as a result of consuming sugar, processed foods, and trans fats. This is non-alcoholic fatty liver disease (NAFLD). It can progress to non-alcoholic steatohepatitis (NASH). Fatty liver from high alcohol consumption is called alcoholic steatohepatitis (ASH). Regardless of the cause of fatty liver disease, it may progress to cirrhosis of the liver, a disease that has no cure.

If you have fatty liver disease you should avoid eating:

Dairy

Hydrogenated/ processed oils

Trans fats

High fructose corn syrup

Agave

Artificial sweeteners

Processed and refined carbohydrates

High fructose fruits (bananas, pineapple, watermelon, mango)

Here's another quiz to help assess how well your digestive system is functioning.

Do you have or experience:

1. __ Indigestion, burping, bloating or lethargic immediately after meals
2. __ Heartburn or acid reflux symptoms
3. __ Undigested food in stool
4. __ Feel like skipping breakfast, overall low appetite
5. __ Sense of excess fullness after meals
6. __ Nausea in evenings
7. __ Proteins or complex meals hard to digest (mix of proteins and carbs)
8. __ History of parasites
9. __ Fungus or yeast infections
10. __ Coating on tongue
11. __ Anemia, unresponsive to iron
12. __ Cramping in lower abdominal region
13. __ Irritable bowel or mucous colitis
14. __ Constipation, stools hard or difficult to pass
15. __ Less than one bowel movement a day
16. __ Pain under right side of rib cage, or between shoulder blades
17. __ Easily intoxicated or hung over if you were to drink wine
18. __ Loose stools with fatty foods, fat in stools (shiny, floating)
19. __ Dry skin, itchy feet or skin peels on feet
20. __ Stomach upset by fatty or fried foods

If you any of these symptoms more than once each week, see a doctor. These can be sign of serious problems that should be treated by a professional.

Numbers 1-7 indicate Hypochlorhydria- too little stomach acid

Numbers 8-11 indicate dysbiosis or an unbalanced microbiome

Numbers 12-15 indicate problems in your lower digestive tract

Numbers 16-20 indicate problems with your gallbladder or liver

If the checklist indicates that your digestive system is not working at its optimum level, there are steps you can take.

To increase the level of hydrochloric acid:

Bitters have long been used as a digestive aid. They can be found in health food stores and some supermarkets. Though they are classified as safe to use, the general recommendation is not to take them if you are pregnant or nursing, or if you have peptic ulcers. Bitters should be mixed with water and taken before meals. Mix 1 teaspoon with 5 teaspoons of water.

Apple cider vinegar can also helpful in increasing the acidity in the stomach. It should be mixed in water 1 tablespoon to ¼ cup of water. This should also be taken before meals containing protein. If this burns your stomach, then you most likely do not have low stomach acid.

To heal the small intestine:

Leaky gut is when your small intestine has been damaged. This stops your intestines from performing its most important task as gatekeeper. There are two things you can do, eliminate foods that are harming you and increase foods that can heal you.

One of the most healing foods you can eat is bone broth. Bone broth has a wealth of collagen, which is a protein found in our bodies that decreases as we age. Collagen is found in our teeth, skin, hair, joints and in our organs. Consuming collagen can improve the way we look and feel.

Bone broth is a traditional food that has been eaten for at least two thousand years. It remains a staple in most cultures, with the exception of the U.S. It was regularly consumed up to a generation ago, and it is making a come-back.

Bone broth is made by slowly simmering the bones of any kind of animal, bird or fish. Bigger beef bones can simmer up to 3 days. Smaller bones from chicken or fish can simmer up to 24 hours. Vegetables are also cooked in the broth to add antioxidants and vitamins.

It's important to choose bones from animals that grazed freely, and were not treated with hormones and antibiotics, and to choose fish that is not high in mercury.

To make a Chicken Bone Broth:

1 chicken carcass
2 carrots
2 celery stalks
2 medium onions
2 garlic cloves
1 Tbs. sea salt
2 bay leaves
1 Tbs. herbs de province
¼ cup vinegar
2 quarts water +/-

Place the carcass in a large stock pot with enough water to cover. Bring to a boil, skimming off the white foam from the top of the stock as it approaches boiling, then reduce the heat so the stock simmers on low. Keep the pot covered.

Add all the additional ingredients and cook for at least 6 and up 24 hours. This can be done on the stove top, or in a crock pot set on low. Add more water as the water evaporates, keeping the bones covered.

Strain through a fine-mesh strainer. If you are not going to be using the stock immediately, chill it as quickly as possible. Cover the stock after it has completely cooled and keep refrigerated for up to 3 days, or freeze for up to 3 months.

To keep the colon healthy:

A healthy colon requires fiber. A diet high in fiber is important for two reasons; it improves stool motility and it feeds the microflora within the colon. Using products such as Beano, which provide enzymes to digest food that can cause gas, also reduces the amount fiber that the colon needs to stay healthy.

Mucilaginous herbs such as slippery elm improves stool motility and enhances colon flora. Herbs that increase the strength of the colon wall include grape seed extract, and hawthorn.

Eating fermented foods and including prebiotic foods in your diet can help maintain a healthy microbiome. Fermented foods include yogurt, kefir, kimchi, sauerkraut, kombucha, kvass, wine and beer. Prebiotics include asparagus, bananas, garlic, honey, onions, and legumes.

Cabbage is extremely beneficial for the digestive tract. This easy ferment will keep in your refrigerator for up to four months.

Fermented Red Cabbage

8 cups shredded cabbage
1 cup chopped onion
1 Tbs. caraway seeds, or mustard seeds
1 Tbs. salt
4 Tbs. whey

Mix all ingredients in a bowl and pound with mallet to release juices for 5- 10 minutes. Place in a wide mouth, 2 quart mason jar. Press down firmly so that the cabbage is below 1" from the top of the jar and juices cover the cabbage. Leave on a counter top for three days then place in refrigerator.

To assist the liver and gallbladder

The liver is a vital organ. If you suspect that your liver is not functioning properly this should be checked by your physician. Problems with the gallbladder can be life-threatening as well. Any suggestions here are made for someone in good health, not for someone with a potentially life-threatening illness.

There are three types of remedies for a liver that is not functioning properly. They are cholagogues, which stimulate bile flow, hepatics, which act to support liver function, and hepatoprotectives, which act to protect the liver. Each of these works to improve the function of the gallbladder as well.

Dandelion is particularly good for the liver. It is both a cholagogue and hepatic. This can be eaten in a salad, or dried and drunk as a tea. While it is generally recognized as safe, it should not be used by anyone with cholecystitis, or any type of bile duct blockage, including gallstones.

Beets also support the liver. They are both hepatic and hepatoprotective. Beets promote regeneration of liver cells, and they are considered detoxifying.

Turmeric, milk thistle, and barberry are also used to support the liver.

I make this salad in the warm months.   When it's cold I take the carrots and beets, add caraway seeds and roast them at 325° for 20 minutes.

Beet Salad

2 shredded beets
4 shredded carrots
½ cup pineapple
1 lemon, juiced
¼ cup currants
1 tsp honey

Combine all ingredients and allow to sit for a few hours so flavors can blend.

Herbs that Act on the Digestive Tract

No one herbal protocol will work for everyone. Each person should consider their own symptoms prior to taking herbal supplements. A registered herbalist can provide additional detail.

There are five classes of herbs that act on the digestion. They are: Carminative, Stomachic, Bitters, Cathartics, and Aperients

Carminatives are used to relieve symptoms of abdominal pain or distension. Peppermint is a type of carminative on which a great deal of research has been conducted. A review of 35 clinical trials found peppermint oil to be among the most effective treatments for irritable bowel syndrome. (15)

Stomachics are used to tone the stomach tissue and improve gastric activity. Ginger is both a stomachic and a carminative. Numerous studies have been conducted to examine the efficacy of ginger on digestive problems. A review of functional foods found that ginger is involved in receptor activities. (10, 66)

Bitters act to stimulate the digestion and appetite. Numerous beneficial digestive properties have been identified as a result of consuming bitters. Recent research has shown that bitters have the ability to stimulate the release of ghrelin, the hormone responsible for stimulating hunger as well. (65)

Cathartics are used to accelerate the movement of food through the digestive tract by increasing the bulk of the feces. Maintaining normal bowel movements is extremely important, not just due to the immediate discomfort, but also for the long-term problems that can develop as a result of too little fiber in the diet.

Aperients purge the digestive tract. Sea Buckthorn is used for its laxative effects. The ability to move food out of the stomach may also assist in the healing of gastric ulcers.

Chapter Three

The Microbiome

The microbiome encompasses the community of microbes that live in your digestive tract. A baby is born sterile, its microbiome begins developing at birth. The infant will continue to develop a diversified microbiome from family, friends, pets, and the environment.

The majority of these microbes live in your colon. Part of their job there is to break down the non-digestible fibers that have passed through your digestive tract. A healthy well-balanced microbiome has the ability to turn these remains into Vitamin K, essential fatty acids, and some B vitamins.

Unfortunately, it is not unusual for people to have the wrong mix of microbes inhabiting their digestive tract. This is due in part to the pervasive use of antibiotics in the food industry. In fact, 80% of antibiotics used in this country are given to live stock. Couple that with our own use of antibiotics, and you can expect to see a much depleted microbiome. Antibiotics kill all microbes, including the ones we need.

We also have diets that do not support good intestinal health. Processed food does not feed your healthy microbes. Sugar feeds bacteria, which moves right into the void left behind when the good microbes are killed off.

The effects of an imbalanced microbiome can lead to a state of chronic inflammation affecting not only internal organs, tendons and joints, but can even lead to the development of cancer. Research has supported the impact of the microbiome on numerous physiological, biochemical, and psychological functions. It has been implicated in the development of obesity, metabolic syndrome, diabetes, and endocrine dysfunctions. (1, 17, 19)

Research on the relationship between the enteric nervous system and and its effect on mood, and the functioning of the central nervous system is proceeding at a rapid pace. From 2007 to 2012 there were only 47 articles published on this topic. But in the past five years there were over 500 articles listed on Pubmed.gov.

The enteric nervous system surrounds the gastrointestinal system, it is also known as the "second brain". This system is populated by an array of sensors, immune cells and vast variety of microbes. There is a nerve that runs from the digestive tract to the brain. This vagus nerve is attached at several places along the digestive tract. It is one of the reasons the systemic impact of the microbiome is so extensive. As the communication runs back and forth between the brain and the digestive tract, 20% is from the brain to the digestive tract, 80% runs from the digestive tract to the brain. (29, 39, 43)

Microbes Affect your Mood and Health

There is a growing body of evidence that finds a correlation between the health of the microbiome and its effect on mood, behavior, and memory. Use of antibiotics and eating a diet high in processed food can lead to dysregulation in the microbiome is often seen concurrent with states of anxiety, depression, memory, and concentration impairment. Fortunately we are able to take an unhealthy microbiome and improve it. (29)

Microbes change in response to changes in the diet. This includes microbes that produce inflammation. For example, bacteroidetes carry lipopolysaccharides in their cell walls. Lipopolysaccharides promote inflammation. Some studies indicate that a high fat diet can decrease the amount of bacteroidetes in the colon. This of course would be a diet high in healthy fats. (19, 35, 41)

Prebiotics and probiotics can have an effect on the metabolic processes within the microbiome. Research is ongoing in the effort to discover how best to influence the complex relationship between the individual, their microbiome, and the food and nutrients consumed. A great place to start would be to limit, or even better, to eliminate processed foods, sugar, and trans fats.

An organic, whole food diet can be supplemented with probiotics and fermented foods. Research has found that consuming fermented milk is associated with changes to midbrain activity, which processes emotion and sensation. Women who consumed fermented milk showed differences in resting brain activity and improved ability in task performance. Fermented milk includes yogurt, cheese and kefir. These are each fermented with different types of microbes. (63)

The food we eat is converted by intestinal microbes into bioactive compounds that affect your health. Prebiotics and probiotics can modulate the immune system in the intestine, actually improving your immune function. The production of short-chain fatty acids is one of the best examples of the way the microbiome works in concert with your immune system.

Research has demonstrated that butyrate and acetate, two short-chain fatty acids produced by the microbiome, are intimately involved with immune response. Butyrate improves the function of helper T-cells and improves the strength of the intestinal lining. This is important because a damaged intestinal lining, or leaky gut, has been implicated in many types inflammation including autoimmune diseases. Acetate also works to keep the intestinal tract in good health. It does this by reducing the rate of infections. It seems to work particularly well to keep *E. coli* in check. (17, 19, 21)

Microbes Require Proper Feeding

It is important to eat a well-balanced, whole food diet in order to maintain healthy colonies of microbial flora. This is due to the varied nutritional requirements of each genus of microbe. If we think in terms of our own nutritional requirements and the consequences of not eating right, we can begin to understand microbial requirements.

For instance, if I ate a diet that was devoid of Vitamin C, I would become more susceptible to colds, my gums would begin to bleed, I would bruise easily and I would eventually develop scurvy. This is because Vitamin C is an antioxidant, and it is a source of collagen. So I would become unhealthy with a lack of Vitamin C. My microbes become unhealthy without prebiotics. Consider prebiotics as microbe food.

Prebiotics of various types are found as natural components in milk, honey, fruits, and vegetables, such as onion, garlic, artichoke, banana, and barley. Asparagus, beets, chicory, tomato, and rye are sources of fructooligosaccharides (FOS).

FOS do not breakdown during digestion. They are instead metabolized or eaten by beneficial microbes and they create short chain fatty acids. Having FOS in your diet has also been shown to increase mineral absorption, and to decrease serum cholesterol and triacylglycerol.

Some microbes, like *Lactobacillus acidophilus* have been studied extensively. This probiotic, which is commonly found in yogurt, has been found to help regulate both diarrhea and constipation, IBS, allergies, eczema, allergies, and it appears to improve immune function. But it needs prebiotics to do these wonderful things. It eats FOS and Isomaltulose.

Isomaltulose is a new candidate as a prebiotic. It naturally occurs in honey, sugarcane juice, and its products such as food-grade molasses. It is not found in refined sugar.

Galactooligosaccharides (GOS) and raffinose oligosaccharides are also prebiotics. Galactooligosaccharides are found naturally in human and bovine milk. Seeds of legumes, lentils, peas, beans, chickpeas, and mustard are rich in raffinose oligosaccharides.

Eating Fermented Foods Increases Healthy Microbes

Probiotic foods help to diversify the balance of microbial species, thereby strengthening your microbiome. Miso has more than 160 bacterial strains along with protein, B-complex vitamins, antioxidants, and it has Vitamin C, carotenoids, chlorophyll, fiber and enzymes.

Making your own fermented foods like kimchi or kombucha is very easy, and less costly than buying them already prepared. Homemade yogurt has 100 billion microbes per serving. That's 100 times more than the 1 billion found in one serving of commercial yogurt.

Kefir is another fermented milk product. It is made by souring milk with a large number and variety of beneficial bacteria and yeast. These strains are able to stay in the digestive tract and help to balance the microbial flora. Yogurt's beneficial microbes don't stay in the digestive tract as long as those found in kefir.

Other fermented foods include sauerkraut (not from a can), buttermilk, tempeh, and pickles. In fact, you can ferment just about any vegetable. There are numerous videos and books on the subject. I highly recommend the book Nourishing Traditions by Sally Fallon, which has many traditional recipes.

Supplementing with Probiotics

Because of the abundance of antibiotics in our livestock, most people could benefit from additional probiotics in their diet. If eating fermented food does not appeal to you, you could take probiotic supplements. As an everyday supplement, take a probiotic with 10 billion colony-forming units (CFUs) per day. These are available in capsules.

If you have just finished a course of antibiotics, supplement with 20-30 billion CFUs per day for at least one month. While you are taking antibiotics, *Saccharomyces boulardii*, a beneficial yeast, can be used to keep digestive problems at bay. Antibiotics target bacteria, not yeast, so *S. boulardii* can survive the antibiotics. Always consult your health care provider before starting a supplementation regimen.

When purchasing probiotics, look for freeze-dried capsules. Freeze-drying sends the microorganisms into hibernation, assuring the best quality. They can be found in the refrigerator section of a whole foods market or health food store. Keep your probiotics in the refrigerator, though a few days at room temperature will not destroy them.

Take probiotics with food, especially foods that are high in fructooligosaccharides (FOS), Galactooligosaccharides (GOS) and raffinose oligosaccharides. These will all work well to feed the microbes.

Don't take your probiotics with stomach acid suppressants or calcium carbonates like Rolaids and Tums. Stomach acid improves the environment for the microbes. This assists the microbes in reaching their destination, the small intestine and colon.

Adults and children benefit from a wide variety of microbes. Strains to look for include lactobacillus and bifidobacteria species, as well *S. boulardii* yeast. Lactobacillus are native to the small intestine and bifidobacteria reside in the colon.

A special strain of bifidobacteria, *Bifidobacterium infantis*, is best suited for babies. The easiest way to give probiotics to infants is to apply the probiotic powder to the nipple of the nursing mother.

Easy Ferments

Kombucha

8 organic black tea bags
1 cup of sugar
1 gallon of filtered water
2 cups of starter kombucha tea
1 SCOBY per fermentation jar

To prepare:

Avoid prolonged contact with stainless steel or metal. Be sure to wash hands and surfaces often.

Bring 1 gallon of filtered water to a boil, add the sugar and stir until it dissolves. Add the tea bags and steep until the water has cooled. Add the starter tea. Transfer to a 1 gallon glass jar and add the SCOBY. Cover the mouth of the jar with several layers of cheesecloth or paper towel. Leave to ferment out of direct sunlight in a warm space (ideal 75F) for 7-10 days. If it is colder, it will take longer to ferment.

Kombucha can be served after the initial fermentation. It can also be double-fermented. Add fruit or herbs and leave out for 3 more days then refrigerate.

Beet-Fruit Kvass

1 medium beet, sliced fine
1 apple, washed and chopped coarsely
1 handful of berries, fresh or frozen
1 Tbs. sea salt
¼ cup whey
1 teaspoon of grated ginger
Water to fill

Place ingredients in a two-quart wide mouth ball jar and fill to the shoulder of the jar with pure water, leaving one inch space from the top. Seal tightly. Ferment for 2 -5 days out of direct sunlight.

When done, store in refrigerator. Drink diluted with water, or drink about 2 oz. per day, undiluted.

NOTE: Kvass may be made from any vegetables or combination of vegetables and fruits and berries, or just fruit and berries.

Part Two

Chapter Four

Inflammation

Inflammation is a normal response to injury. This might be a physical injury, or micro-tears in our blood vessels. In either case the body responds by increasing the blood supply to the injured area and sending monocytes to begin repair work and phagocytes to clean up the debris.

We run into problems when this process is chronic. For instance high blood pressure causes constant tears in the blood vessels, which will begin to narrow due to the ongoing repair work within the body. This can affect the brain as well as the heart. The same veins that bring oxygen and nutrients to the heart are also supplying the brain.

Eating foods that are high in saturated fats and trans fats can cause fat cells to become inflamed and can worsen conditions such as arthritis and heart disease. These foods include dairy and animal fats, processed food and fast-food.

The standard American diet has too little omega-3 and too much omega 6 fats. The body needs both of these fats to be in better balance. Omega 3s are found in salmon, sardines, walnuts and flaxseeds. Omega 6s are found in refined oils, fast foods, and processed foods.

Some other factors contributing to inflammation:

Not getting enough exercise will further exacerbate these problems. Fat is pro-inflammatory, while exercising muscles will reduce inflammation and improve insulin sensitivity.

Eating a diet that is high in sugar will cause the release of pro-inflammatory cytokines, which cause pain and inflammation.

Preservatives like MSG, which can be found in many processed foods leads to increased inflammation.

Food sensitivities such as the gluten found in wheat and casein found in dairy can both be triggers for inflammation. An elimination diet can help identify food sensitivities.

Reducing Inflammation

Most people think of the aging process as the inevitable march toward physical and cognitive decline, but that doesn't have to be the case. Numerous studies find that people eating a largely plant based diet have lower rates of neurological impairment, heart disease, arthritis, and even cancer. This is due in part to these people having lower levels in inflammation throughout their bodies. (48, 66, 68)

A cross sectional study of 1898 women aged 18-75 years from the Twins UK registry found that a diet high in flavanones, anthocyanins, and flavonols, led to a decrease in arterial stiffness, central blood pressure, and atherosclerosis. Where are these mysterious compounds found? Flavanones are in parsley, peppers, apples and watermelon. Anthocyanins can be found in berries, bananas, pears, cabbage and garbanzo beans. There are flavonols in onions, tomatoes, sweet potatoes, and quinoa. (34)

Green smoothies are not a youth elixir, but a high-fiber plant based diet does lead to better health. People who consume high levels of fiber carry fewer toxins. This is because toxins bind to fiber and the body is then able to excrete them.

Recommendations for dietary changes include increasing foods with beneficial antioxidants, phytochemicals and nutraceuticals and decreasing foods known to create inflammation. The standard American diet is fraught with the ingredients that should be avoided, and is low in nutrient density.

A closer look at the specific nutrients that have been cited in studies finds that a diet high in fruit and Vitamin C provides strong protective factors. Vitamin C can be found in citrus fruits, berries, kiwi, broccoli, and peas. It is also one of the building blocks of collagen, which is the most abundant protein in the body.

Beta- and gamma-tocopherols have been investigated as part of the diet. Beta- and gamma-tocopherols are the main plant forms of Vitamin E, but they are generally not found in supplements. Beta-tocopherols tend to be more difficult for the body to absorb and are not as well-studied as gamma-tocopherols. Gamma-tocopherols can be found in black walnuts, sesame seeds, pecans, pistachios, English walnuts, flaxseeds, and pumpkin seeds.

Foods rich in polyphenols have been noted for their anti-inflammatory properties. They are found in many fruits and vegetables. Polyphenols are also found in green tea, dark chocolate, berries, flaxseed, olives, apples, spinach, red wine, and grape juice.

High Blood Pressure

High blood pressure or hypertension is the process of the arteries becoming narrowed. It begins when there are tiny tears to the endothelial layer of cells, which line the veins and arteries. As the body rebuilds the damaged areas scar tissue adheres to the tears. As this process continues the cells become engorged, further narrowing the arteries.

However, the development of atherosclerosis is more complex than the development of plaque on the artery walls. The progression can be affected by stress, toxins, and infections and viruses. High blood pressure responds well to a change in the diet.

I thought it would be helpful to take a closer look at the ways in which food can have an effect on chronic health conditions, a neurological disorder and an infectious disease. Here are some compounds in common foods that work to reduce high blood pressure:

Resveratrol (Stilbene): Found in wine, grapes, blueberries, bilberries, dark chocolate and peanuts. One of the best known anti-inflammatory foods, resveratrol is reported to cross the blood-brain barrier, which means it may be able to help protect your brain and nervous system. It is also known for protecting your cells from free radical damage, lowering your blood pressure, keeping your heart healthy, and improving elasticity in your blood vessels.

Catechins (Flavonoid): Found in high concentrations in green tea and in lower concentrations in black tea. They are also found in berries and dark chocolate. They may reduce the risk of stroke, heart disease, and they lower cholesteryl.

Procyanidins (Polyphenol): Found in red wine, dark chocolate, apples, cranberries, these have been noted for improving cardiovascular health.

Astaxanthin (Carotenoid): Found in salmon, lobster, crab, krill, shrimp, and algae. Its anti-inflammatory properties may make it useful in maintaining heart, brain, and joint health.

Lycopene (Carotenoid): Found in tomatoes, watermelon, and pink grapefruit, it may reduce the risk of cancer, heart disease, and may also reduce LDL cholesterol ("bad" cholesterol).

The three main forms of omega 3 Fatty Acids are eicosapentaenoic acid (EPA), docosahexaenoic acid (DHA), and alpha-linolenic acid (ALA). ALA is a short-chain form of Fatty Acid, which is found in plants. EPA and DHA are long-chain forms of omega-3 Fatty Acid. Foods containing Omega-3 Fatty Acids: Oily fish like salmon, halibut, and anchovies contain EPA and DHA. Walnuts, and nut oils, flax seed and flax seed oil, pumpkin seeds, and canola oil contain ALA. EPA, DHA and ALA are all essential fatty acids, which your body needs but cannot make on its own. These may reduce inflammation, lower the risk of cardiovascular disease, and improve cognitive function and joint inflammation.

Oleocanthal: This phenylethanoid is among 36 phenolic compounds found in olive oil. It is being investigated for its ability to reduce inflammation, for its antioxidant status, and for its antimicrobial activity. (49)

Arthritis

Osteoarthritis is the leading cause of disability in America and the rate of incidence is rising. This debilitating disease features symptoms that include pain, stiffness, and loss of function in the affected joints. It is most often seen in the hands, feet, knees, and spine.

A diet low in saturated fat and high in phyto-nutrients is generally recommended. Studies have found links between a healthy whole food diet and improved symptoms in people with osteoarthritis. Foods rich in polyphenols and high in fruit and Vitamin C provided the strongest protective factor. (35)

Complementary and alternative treatments for osteoarthritis can have fewer side-effects than those seen in traditional western treatment recommendations. Glucosamine has been supported by numerous studies, as has curcumin, which is a derived from turmeric. Both have been used as anti-inflammatories. (31)

Helpful Herbs

No one herbal protocol will work for everyone. Each person should consider their own symptoms prior to taking herbal supplements. A registered herbalist can provide additional detail.

Ginger is best known for its positive effects on the digestion; however, it has numerous other applications, among which is its effect on inflammation. Ginger is an anti-inflammatory and analgesic. Fresh ginger can be grated into food or drinks and can be safely consumed once or twice daily.

Nettles are an herb with anti-inflammatory properties. Nettles can be purchased dried in bulk or in prepackaged tea bags. A tea can be prepared once or twice daily. Once the tea has been made, the leftover nettle leaves can be added to soups or stews. It is very nutrient dense with high levels of potassium, calcium, phenolic acid, and carotenoids.

Turmeric, or more specifically its active component curcumin, is an antioxidant and anti-inflammatory with the ability to regulate pro-inflammatory cytokines. Recent studies indicate that it is involved in inflammatory pathways. Eating turmeric will not cause the problems associated with the use of commonly prescribed medications, such as upper and lower gastrointestinal bleeding, and increased cardiovascular risks. (31)

Cat's Claw is an anti-inflammatory. It relieves pain associated with arthritis. It should not be taken during pregnancy, or with blood-thinning or immunosuppressing medications.

Calendula is an anti-inflammatory with wound-healing properties. It acts to provide relief from muscle aches, joint tenderness, while supporting the immune system.

Dandelion is an antioxidant that supports detoxification and relieves chronic rheumatic pain.

Garlic is an antioxidant, antibacterial, antifungal, and antihypertensive.

Licorice is an anti-inflammatory, antioxidant, antibacterial, antiviral, antifungal, and improves symptoms of fatigue and chronic rheumatic pain. It should not be taken during pregnancy, or in cases of severe kidney or liver disorders.

Migraines

Migraines are intense headaches characterized by a pulsing or throbbing sensation in one area of the head. They are often accompanied by nausea, vomiting, extreme sensitivity to light and sound, and to visual disturbances known as auras.

The pain associated with migraines is often preceded by the sensory warning of these auras, and may include flashes of light, blind spots, and tingling in extremities. Migraine attacks can last for several hours to a few days, evolving in severity throughout their duration. Migraine headaches are caused by excessive dilation of blood vessels in the head. They affect 15-20% of men and 25-30% of women

Due to its complex neurological nature, a multi-faceted approach is often required to successfully mitigate the severity and frequency of migraines.

The primary treatment focus should be:

Elimination of food sensitivities

Optimization of serotonin levels

Enhancement of micronutrient status, specifically magnesium, calcium, Vitamin B2 and Vitamin B6.

Balance blood sugar. Hypoglycemia can trigger a migraine. Avoid refined carbohydrates and eat meals at regular intervals to avoid peaks and drops in your blood sugar.

Avoid food allergens and irritants. Food sensitivities may contribute to a migraine. Therefore if you are lactose intolerant, avoiding dairy may provide relief. Avoid gluten and other potential food antigens if you have known sensitivities to them.

Common foods that are known to trigger headaches are artificial sweeteners, birth control pills, caffeine, citrus fruits, salt, lactose, monosodium glutamate (MSG) and food additives

If you are unsure of a food sensitivity, conduct an elimination diet of one suspected food at a time for at least two weeks. A better approach is to remove all possible food triggers from your diet, then reintroduce one food at a time and note your reactions.

Note potential triggers. Journal to help identify your particular triggers. Stress plays a large role in migraines. Studies have found that meditation can reduce symptoms of migraines.

Improve gastrointestinal health. The majority of serotonin is produced in the GI tract. Imbalances in gut bacteria or inflammation may impair serotonin synthesis and activity.

Stay hydrated. Dehydration is a common cause of headaches. Try to consume half your body weight in ounces daily (e.g., a 150 lb. person should consume 75 fluid ounces of liquid). Incorporate coconut water into a smoothies and beverage rotation. Eat hydrating fruits and veggies such as celery, cucumber, and watermelon.

Increase the intake of foods that are rich in magnesium and calcium. These minerals help prevent and relieve headaches. Such foods include a variety of fruits and vegetables, brown rice, wheat bran, wheat germ and soy beans.

Avoid eating this:

Foods that are high in amines, specifically histamine and tyramine, have been linked to migraines. These foods contain vasoactive compounds that can trigger migraines in sensitive individuals by causing blood vessels to expand. High histamine foods include:

Seafood: shellfish or fin fish, fresh, frozen, smoked or canned

Eggs

Processed, cured, smoked and fermented meats such as lunch meat, bacon, sausage, salami, pepperoni

All fermented milk products, including most cheeses, yogurt, buttermilk, kefir

Citrus fruits including oranges, grapefruit, lemons, lime

Fermented foods such as sauerkraut, kombucha, pickles, relishes, fermented soy products, etc.

Tomatoes, including ketchup, tomato sauces

Artificial food colors and preservatives

Spices such as cinnamon, chili powder, cloves, anise, nutmeg, curry powder, cayenne

Beverages like tea, alcohol, chocolate, cocoa, and cola drinks

Vinegar and foods containing vinegar such as pickles, relishes, ketchup, and prepared mustard

Sulfites are also problematic. A salt of sulfurous acid is in many processed foods and alcoholic beverages, especially red wine. Eat organic whole foods in order to avoid these.

Food additives such as monosodium glutamate (MSG), aspartame (NutraSweet), and nitrites should also be avoided.

Eat more of this:

Foods that inhibit platelet aggregation like cod liver oil, garlic, onions, and ginger

High-serotonin precursors (tryptophan) such as spirulina, pork, and turkey

High-potassium foods like baked potato with skin, banana, spinach, and winter squash

Magnesium-rich foods including edamame, pumpkin seeds, swiss chard, soybeans

Calcium-rich foods like sesame seeds, collard greens, turnip greens

Non-citrus fruits such as Cherries, Cranberries, Pears, Prunes

Hydrating foods including coconut water, watermelon, celery and lots of water

Also include spicy peppers which have analgesic or pain relieving properties

Herbs and Supplements

No one herbal protocol will work for everyone. Each person should consider their own symptoms prior to taking herbal supplements. A registered Herbalist can provide additional detail.

Feverfew* has been used for hundreds of years for treatment of headaches. It is known for its anti-inflammatory properties and ability to prevent migraines. It can be taken as a dried leaf, fresh plant tincture, or dried plant tincture.

Ginkgo is an antioxidant and anti-inflammatory with vascular, anti-platelet and anticoagulant effects. It alters neurotransmitters and acts as a neuro-protector. CAUTION: While ginkgo appears to be safe in healthy individuals, it does have numerous drug interactions, such as the potential to increase bleeding risk when taking warfarin. Ginkgo can be taken as a dried herb or fluid extract.

Ginger* has anti-inflammatory and antihistamine actions, and affects platelet aggregation. It has the ability to improve signs of nausea, which is often seen in people who experience migraines. CAUTION: High doses of ginger are not recommended for children under the age of six. It has interactions with anti-platelet drugs and warfarin due to its anti-platelet effects. Ginger can be used in liquid extract, dried root or infusion of fresh ginger in boiling water.

*Should not be taken during pregnancy

Other herbs and supplements of note:

Purple butterbur*, which should not be taken during pregnancy or lactation, can be helpful for use in reducing headache pain especially due to tension headaches.

Fish oil may assist in the reduction of migraines through its effect on platelet aggregation.

Magnesium functions to maintain the tone of blood vessels, prevents over-excitability of nerve cells and is a critical nutrient in carbohydrate metabolism.

Vitamin B6 is necessary in order to produce histamine-lowering enzymes.

Vitamin B2 (Riboflavin) can help reduce the incidence of migraines. Riboflavin improves your brain's energy levels and helps protect brain cells.

CoQ10 is a major source of energy production in the whole body. It is also important for blood vessel health and is a powerful antioxidant, which protects your body from free radicals.

Calcium helps to control muscle and nerve functioning as well as to build strong bones and teeth.

Lyme Disease

The Infectious Disease Society of America and the Center for Disease Control hold the traditional view on Lyme disease, recognizing the typically seen symptoms:

A bullseye rash

A fever

A headache

Muscle and joint aches

A stiff neck

Fatigue

Lyme Literate Physicians and the International Lyme and Associated Disease Society hold alternative viewpoints with a broader set of recognized symptoms. These include:

Fatigue

Night sweats

Sore throat

Swollen glands

Arthritis

Chest pain

Sleep disturbances

Problems concentrating

Back pain

Blurred vision

Vertigo

Tinnitus and more...

Lyme disease is often seen with co-infections. These include Babesia, Ehrlichiosis and Bartonella. Secondary infections include Mycoplasma, Candida, Cytomegaly virus, and Epstein-Barr virus.

Because of the complexity of the disease and due to the possibility of co-infections and secondary infections, a three-pronged approach can be helpful in restoring health. The Lyme disease must be attached, while supporting the immune system and killing off residual neurotoxins.

Food is foundational in supporting the immune system. The body must rest, and stress must be decreased to regain strength. The microbiome must be reestablished following antibiotic treatment. Probiotics can be taken, and should be supplemented with fermented food. Herbs can be used to both assist in fighting the disease and co-infections and in support of the immune system.

Foods that are particularly helpful during the recovery from Lyme disease include:

Nutrient-dense, unprocessed, whole foods

Quality oils such as coconut, olive, sesame, flax, and ghee

Raw and cooked non-starchy vegetables including leafy greens

Grass-fed, organic meats and poultry

Wild-caught fish

Fresh herbs and spices especially garlic, ginger, and turmeric

Non-gluten containing grains including quinoa, buckwheat and millet

Nuts and seeds including chia, flax, and hemp seeds

Legumes

Sea vegetables

Fruits especially low-glycemic fruits like berries, and citrus fruits

Starchy vegetables like carrots, rutabagas, beets, and carrots

Sauerkraut and other traditionally fermented foods

These foods are not helpful and should be avoided:

Refined carbohydrates and gluten-containing grains and flour

White rice

Cereals

Dairy including cheese, cream, milk, butter

Sugar

Conventionally raised meat and processed meats

Foods that may be high in mold or yeast such as peanuts, dried fruits, alcohol

High sugar fruits and fruit juices

Possible or known food sensitivities such as wheat, dairy, soy, corn

Hydrogenated and processed vegetable oils, such as soy, canola, corn

Some helpful herbs include:

No one herbal protocol will work for everyone. Each person should consider their own symptoms prior to taking herbal supplements. A registered Herbalist can provide additional detail.

Andrographis*: Anti-inflammatory, antipyretic (reduces fever), antibacterial, choleretic, mild immunomodulant, stimulates immune system, and can decreases pathogenic microbes.

Burdock: A diuretic, antimicrobial, antidyscratic (blood purifier), with wound healing properties. Reduces chronic rheumatic pain. Supports detoxification helping to remove microbes from system.

Cat's Claw*: An anti-inflammatory, immunomodulant. Works well to decrease frequent relapse accompanied by fatigue. Relieves pain associated with arthritis. Should not be taken with blood thinning, or immunosupressing medications.

Calendula: An anti-inflammatory, antimicrobial, Immunomodulants (modifies the way the immune system works), with wound-healing properties. It acts to provide relief from muscle aches, joint tenderness, while supporting the immune system.

Dandelion: An antioxidant, antidyscratic (blood purifier). Supports detoxification and relieves chronic rheumatic pain.

Garlic: An antioxidant, antibacterial, antifungal, anthelmintic (kills parasitic worms), antihypertensive.

Ginger: An anti-inflammatory, analgesic, cholagogue, cardio tonic, antibacterial, antifungal.

Japanese Knotweed: An anti-inflammatory, demulcent (forms soothing film over mucus membrane inflamed tissue).

Licorice*: An anti-inflammatory, antioxidant, antibacterial, antiviral, antifungal, improves symptoms of fatigue, and chronic rheumatic pain. Should not be taken in cases of severe kidney or liver disorders.

Sarsaparilla: A diuretic, anti-inflammatory, antifungal, anti-inflammatory, antidyscratic (blood purifier).

*Should not be taken during pregnancy

Chapter Five

Detoxification

The topic of detoxing has been called into question in recent years. Some proponents have mislabeled, misled and encouraged misuse of detoxification plans that simply don't work. However, properly used, a detox plan can be a good first step in cleaning up some unhealthy eating patterns, it can assist in identifying food sensitivities, it can improve liver function, and it can remove toxins from the body.

Spring time is a great time to transition to a cleaner diet. During winter the body must work at keeping warm. Therefore, cooked and traditionally preserved foods are eaten as a ready source of fuel. During spring our bodies don't have this need. This is also the time of year when bitter greens, which are excellent detoxifiers, begin to grow.

Detox plans can vary from simply eating a cleaner more plant-based diet to a chelation to clear heavy metals from the system. The latter should only be conducted following tests with findings of high levels of lead or mercury and under professional supervision. Between these two extremes there are liquid fasts, raw food plans, along with teas, herbs, and supplements. The goals of these plans are generally the same: to purge the body of toxins.

The body has several ways to rid itself of toxins:

The respiratory system

The digestive system

The lymphatic system

The excretory system

The urinary system

The skin and body membranes

The endocrine system is also indirectly involved as the endocrine cells throughout the digestive tract are involved in the entire digestive process.

When thinking about detoxification, the lungs may not immediately come to mind. However, they are responsible for the removal of gaseous waste from the body. Without the respiratory system's excretory properties we would die from the build-up of carbon dioxide in our cells.

The digestive system clears toxins from the body on a regular basis. An extreme example of this is the effect from a bout of food poisoning. This is detoxification at work. Less dramatically, stomach acid and various types of cells throughout the digestive tract work to protect the body from pathogens and to excrete harmful bacteria along with other waste. The liver is the most important organ for detoxification and is extremely important in the digestive process. In addition to its numerous metabolic roles, the liver detoxifies drugs and alcohol, and its phagocytic cells ingest and excrete bacteria.

The lymphatic system also encounters toxins on a regular basis. It kicks into high gear following illness or injury, providing a complex defense system to heal injuries and destroy pathogens. As part of the body's immune system, it works by employing lymphocytes and phagocytes to attack and remove microorganisms, foreign cells, and cancerous cells. It is also responsible for the day-to-day drainage of waste from the cells.

The excretory system's function is to remove waste, including toxins from the body. The urinary system works in concert with the circulatory system to remove waste from the blood. The kidneys are also responsible for maintaining the proper fluid balance of the blood, the acid-base balance, and electrolyte balance.

In addition to protecting the body from the environment, the skin and body membranes act as both an intricate warning system through its connection to the sensory cortex, and as part of the excretory system through its distribution of sweat glands. Sweat serves to regulate the body's temperature and it secretes acidic chemical barriers to deter the growth of bacteria.

Toxin Quiz

Do/are you:

1. __ Rarely break out into a sweat
2. __ Use aluminum cooking equipment
3. __ Have mercury amalgams
4. __ Feel "wired" or anxious, have heart palpitations, sweat, or feel dizzy after consuming caffeine
5. __ Frequently exposed to solvents and chemicals at work or at home
6. __ Urinate small amounts of dark urine only a few times a day
7. __ Eat large fish (sword fish, tuna, shark, tilefish) more than once a week
8. __ Use tobacco products
9. __ Use lawn or garden chemicals
10. __ Live in a large urban or industrial area
11. __ Drink less than 4 cups water a day
12. __ Have strong body odor
13. __ Eat "fast-food" more than 2 times a week
14. __ Have your clothes dry-cleaned
15. __ Drink unfiltered tap, well or bottled water? (Circle one)

If you checked off one or two of these you are at moderate risk, and should consider making some changes to your lifestyle.

If you checked off more than five of these you are at high risk, and should consider a detoxification plan.

If you checked off more than ten of these you are at extremely high risk and should speak to your doctor.

Improving Detoxification Pathways

The Respiratory System

The respiratory is generally not impacted by toxins unless you smoke or are exposed to chemicals or fumes. This system certainly slows down when you have phlegm or mucus from a cold or bronchitis. There are a few things you can take to help your respiratory system. Garlic is an excellent antioxidant, antibacterial, and antifungal. It can be helpful in fighting many infections. It works in the lungs because allicin, which is the active ingredient, is excreted through the lungs when you breathe. It's one of the reasons we get garlic breath.

Eucalyptus is also excreted through the lungs. It is antimicrobial, and anti-inflammatory. It can be drunk as a tea. Of course if you have a persistent cough, or pain when you breathe, you should see your physician.

The Digestive System

The Digestive System was covered in the previous section. Having the proper level of hydrochloric acid is important for detoxifying, or killing dangerous microbes. There are steps you can take to increase levels of hydrochloric acid. Following those recommendations will not just help you break down food, it will improve your digestive detoxification as well.

The same is true of the microbiome. The content of your microbial colonies can contribute to your overall toxic load, depending on the types of microbes inhabiting your digestive tract. The food you eat can help or hurt your microbes leading to either a healthy microbiome or one that is compromised by dysbiosis, which is an imbalance in the flora of the microbiome. Follow the recommendations in the previous section to improve your microbiome.

The liver is a vital organ. If you suspect that your liver is not functioning properly this should be checked by your physician. Otherwise if you just feel like you'd like to give your liver beneficial foods, follow the recommendations in the previous section.

The Lymphatic System

It is not unusual for the lymph nodes to become inflamed during the course of a cold or other virus. They are part of your body's immune response and can become enlarged when they are working to clear an infection. Typically the swelling will subside after a few days.

If you are very uncomfortable you can try drinking calendula tea, which is anti-inflammatory, and antimicrobial. Echinacea has been used to assist in both strengthening lymphatic function and drainage. If your lymph nodes remain swollen see your physician.

The Excretory System, the Urinary System

Increasing water consumption is vital during the detoxification process. A minimum of two to three quarts should be drunk. This will help to remove toxins from your body.

Parsley can be used to flush the kidneys, and will increase urination. This should not be done by anyone with kidney stones. Asparagus is also a diuretic and it is soothing to the urinary tract. Yarrow and uva ursi are also soothing diuretics that can be taken as herbal teas.

The Excretory System, the Skin and Body Membranes

Skin needs to sweat in order to purge toxins. This can be accomplished externally by using a sauna or hot tub. Sweat can also be induced through exercise. Any type of activity that raises your body temperature is beneficial. Food can also cause the body to perspire. They are called diaphoretics and they include many types of hot peppers. These can be used fresh or dried. Ginger and peppermint can also be used as diaphoretics. This will be most effective when drunk as a hot tea.

General Recommendations for a Cleaner Diet

When looking at your overall eating patterns consider this:

__ What percentage of your diet is raw, this includes fresh fruits and salads?

__ What percentage of your diet freshly is cooked meats or vegetables?

__ What percentage is unprocessed grains?

__ What percentage is from a box, like cereal, breakfast bars and other snacks?

__ What percentage comes from a bag, like bread or instant meals?

__ What percentage of your beverages have sweeteners added?

__ Are there trans fats in your diet?

Which of these look like your current eating pattern?

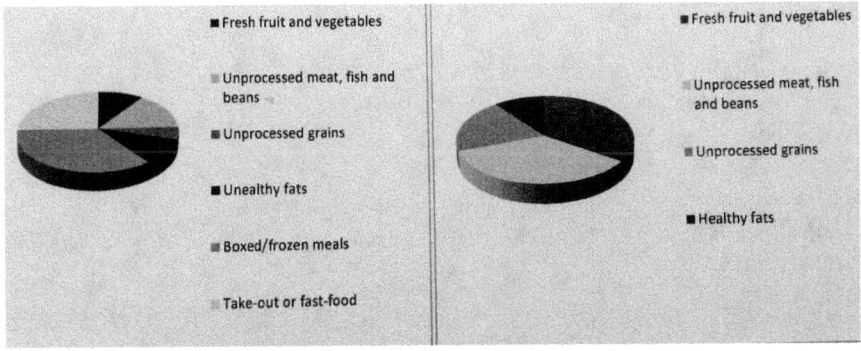

If your eating pattern looks more like the left chart than the right chart, your diet should be improved. The first four categories should make up the bulk of your diet. The more boxed, bagged, processed and sweetened food in your diet, the more health problems you will develop over time.

The excess sodium, unhealthy fats and sweeteners in prepared meals contribute to high blood pressure, elevated cholesterol, heart disease, and diabetes. It is also not uncommon for people who eat these types of foods to feel chronically tired, suffer from headaches, and to suffer from joint pain.

The good news is it is fairly easy to improve your eating patterns. With a little planning you can be on your way to a cleaner eating plan.

Adding fresh juices, smoothies and raw food to your diet is an easy first step to improving your eating patterns. Raw food and salads aid in detoxifying the body. The enzymes present in fresh raw food remains intact. These are the phyto-chemicals that help plants to grow. They are lost once the plants have been cooked.

As you begin to incorporate raw foods to your diet, it is important to remember the basic components of good nutrition. Protein, carbohydrates, and healthy fats are part of a well-balanced diet. You will want to be sure your meals remain balanced. One of my favorite ways to eating my antioxidants is in dips and pesto.

Dandelion-Nettle Pesto

½ cup olive oil
¼ cup fresh dandelion greens
¼ cup dried nettles
¼ cup fresh basil or cilantro
½ cup olive oil
½ cup almonds
2 cloves garlic
1 tsp. salt

Grind the almonds a in food processor. Add the remaining ingredients and blend until smooth. More or less olive oil can be added, and salt can also be adjusted to taste. This can be used as a dip, or it can be poured over rice, or it can be used to top fish or chicken for grilling or baking.

Antioxidants

Antioxidants are naturally occurring substances found in many foods. They are much like vitamins and minerals. Some vitamins, such as Vitamin C, are also antioxidants. Antioxidants fight free radicals and protect cells from oxidative damage, which can lead to disease.

Some of the protective effects of antioxidants are listed here:

Polyphenols fight free radicals, reduce inflammation, and protect the cardiovascular system. There are over 8,000 identified polyphenols, which can be broken into 4 categories: flavonoids, stilbenes, lignans, and phenolic acids.

Lignan intake has been linked to a lower risk of cardiovascular disease, lower rates of cancer and may even help prevent bone loss. They are found in various seeds including flax, pumpkin and sunflower seeds, as well as kale, broccoli and berries.

Flavonoids are broken into six additional classes: anthocyanins, flavan-3-ols, flavonols, flavanones, flavones, and isoflavones.

Anthocyanins are found in red, blue, and purple berries, red and purple grapes, and red wine. These powerful antioxidants are potent free-radical scavengers. They have been studied for their positive effects on reducing blood pressure, improving eyesight, and lowering the rates of neurological diseases. (45)

Flavan-3-ols can be found in apples, berries, grapes, cocoa and tea especially white, green, and oolong. These have been studied most in relation to their ability to lower risks of cardiovascular disease.

Flavonols are also found in tea, as well as onions, scallions, kale, broccoli, apples, berries. There is evidence that they are associated with a reduced risk of stroke and hypertension. (53)

Flavanones are in parsley, thyme, celery, and hot peppers. There is evidence that these antioxidants reduce inflammation. (65)

Flavones can be found in citrus fruit and juices. They are currently being studied for their ability to reduce the effects of oxidative stress. (47)

Isoflavones are phytoestrogens and are found in soybeans, soy foods, and legumes. They have been linked to lower rates of coronary disease. They should only be consumed in non-processed foods.

Stilbenes are best known for resveratrol and piceatannol (tannins), and can be found in wine, grapes, peanuts, cocoa, strawberries, rhubarb, tomatoes, and cranberries. Resveratrol has been linked to a reduction in pro-inflammatory cytokines, which play a role in the development of inflammatory diseases. (66)

Phenolic acids are found in a broad range of plant-based foods, ranging from fruits and vegetables to grains and legumes. The highest concentrations are found in berries, citrus fruits, apples, grapes, cherries, onion, artichokes, rhubarb, red cabbage, buckwheat, oats, coffee, cocoa, red wine, and black and green teas.

Vitamin A: There are two types of Vitamin A. Retinol is found in liver, fish, dairy and eggs, Provitamin A or carotenoids are in carrots, cantaloupe, and squash. Vitamin A is involved in eye and skin health, and neurological function.

Vitamin C: Citrus fruits, peppers, kale, and berries. It improves immune function, mineral absorption, fights free radicals and builds collagen.

Vitamin E: Sunflower seeds, almonds, spinach, beet greens, avocado, improves and protects hair and skin.

Zeaxanthin (Carotenoid): Spinach, kale, and dark leafy greens, and eggs, may minimize the effects of age-related macular degeneration.

Lycopene (Carotenoid): Tomatoes, watermelon, and pink grapefruit. It may reduce the risk of cancer, heart disease, and may also reduce LDL cholesteryl.

Procyanidins (Polyphenol): Red wine, dark chocolate, apples and cranberries have been noted for improving cardiovascular health.

Quercetin (Flavenoid): Apples, grapes and wine work against cancer cells, induce cell death in certain types of cancers, and reduce the release of histamine, providing an anti-inflammatory and antihistamine effect.

Selenium is a mineral with antioxidant properties. It's found in brazil nuts, turkey, mushrooms, fish and eggs. It protects cells from free radical damage.

Sulfur Rich foods: These enhance glutathione production, which is a crucial peptide produced by our bodies. These foods include arugula, cabbage, cauliflower, bok choy, water cress, broccoli, and brussel sprouts. Vitamins B6, B9, B12, and biotin, as well as selenium, also improve the production of glutathione.

Glutathione is involved in numerous functions which include assisting the liver in detoxification. It is a co-factor in several enzymatic processes protecting cells from oxidative damage, and it's involved in immune function.

The benefit of consuming your antioxidants from food, rather than from supplements, is that your body can better regulate the absorption. It's much more difficult to take too much when it's carried in the food you eat. The food also has the added benefit of creating synergy, that is to say that the various constituents in food can boost or blunt the absorption of the nutrients it carries.

Here are a few simple juice recipes. They are made by running these ingredients through a juicer. Alternatively they could be tossed in a high speed blender and turned into a smoothie. To make a creamy smoothie you can add half an avocado or banana to one of these recipes along with some ice. Adding some yogurt or nut butter will make this a complete meal.

Super Juice

1 Pepper
2 Carrots
2 pieces of Kale
2 stalks of Celery
1 small piece of Ginger
1 Beet
1 small clove Garlic

Green Juice

1 Lemon
2 stalks of Celery
1 handful of Spinach
2 pieces of Kale
½ a small Cucumber

Part Three

Chapter Six

Food and Mood

Proper nutrition gives your body the energy you need to do your daily activities, to think clearly, and to have the emotional reserves to handle challenges that might arise. Can you think of a time when you were hungry and it affected your behavior or ability to handle a challenge? This is your body's way of telling you to meet its needs!

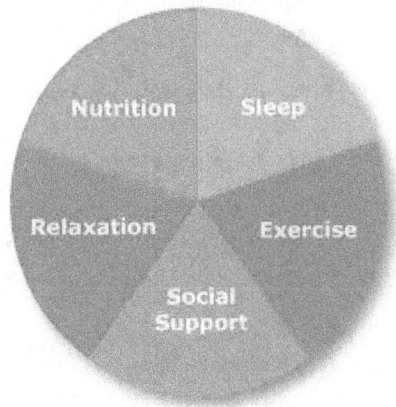

This wheel can help you examine areas of your life you may be neglecting. On a scale of 1-10, with 10 being completely satisfied, rate each area.

It may seem strange to consider these areas in relation to food and mood, but consider that if you aren't getting the sleep you need your body will need more energy, and you will become hungry. If you have no social supports, you may eat out of loneliness. No relaxation may lead to eating because you are anxious. Exercise can actually curtail grazing, and it helps to build muscle and stamina, while burning calories. Finally, feeding your body a nutrient dense diet can help to reduce food cravings.

Food Cravings and Dietary Deficiencies

Food cravings are often spoken of in relation to the type of food you're "in the mood for". You may be seeking comfort in sweet or creamy foods. Or chewing on crunchy foods when feeling stressed. But there are also instances when food cravings can be tied to deficiencies.

When people crave fats they are often deficient in essential fatty acids. Try increasing fatty fish in your diet, add flax seed oil to your salads along with avocados, and consider adding a fish oil supplement to your diet.

You may also be deficient in tyrosine, iodine, folic acid, or your copper/zinc ratio may be out of balance. You may even be suffering from hypothyroidism. If increasing your healthy fats doesn't decrease your fat cravings see your doctor for additional testing.

Salt cravings often point to a magnesium deficiency. Are you also craving chocolate? Same thing, magnesium! Foods high in magnesium include edamame, pumpkin seeds, swiss chard, soybeans, and salmon. You could also take a magnesium supplement.

Cravings for dairy products and baked goods are often an indication that you may have a sensitivity to these very things. Try an elimination diet for a few weeks to see if your dairy and wheat cravings decrease. If you felt no difference after 2 weeks, try adding a probiotic to your diet.

Impact of Unhealthy Food Choices

While there's nothing wrong with giving in and indulging in the occasional treat, constantly eating the following foods can lead to chronic health conditions.

Refined Carbohydrates and Sugar: There's really nothing good to say about these food products. They contribute to high levels of inflammation throughout the body, they are devoid of nutritional value, and they are even tied to increased symptoms of depression.

Artificial Sweeteners: There are numerous studies tying artificial sweeteners to weight gain, tumors, and cancer. However, the scientific community remains divided on the safety of these food additives. In a study on the neurobehavioral effects of aspartame, researchers found that healthy individuals with no history of depression exhibited symptoms of irritable mood and depression, as well as decreased spatial orientation, when they consumed aspartame for just one week. (39)

Trans fats: Trans fats have also been the topic of numerous research studies measuring the correlation between its consumption and its effect on mood. These artificially created fats are not processed in our bodies the same way that natural, healthy fats are. Therefore rather than being a benefit to our brain health, they act as a deterrent causing inflammation, affecting memory and creating a depressed state. (63)

Processed foods: This group of "foods" includes all the negative attributes of the aforementioned groups. Studies have linked diets high in processed foods to erratic behavior, mood swings, depression, and violent outbursts. There are several reasons for this. These foods are metabolized quickly leading to energy peaks and crashes, and diets high in processed foods are tied to vitamin and mineral deficiencies. This lack of vitamins and minerals leads to an inability to produce the chemicals and hormones necessary for proper brain function. (62)

Timing of Meals

It is important to consider the timing of your meals in addition to the content. Your brain requires fuel to run at an optimal level. Struggling with hypoglycemia can be just as challenging as the high glycemic spikes that sugar and refined carbohydrates induce it.

People who suffer from anxiety are particularly affected by hypoglycemia. Consider the symptoms of hypoglycemia:

Confusion

Dizziness

Feeling shaky

Headaches

Irritability

Pounding heart

Pale skin

Sweating

Weakness

Anxiety

To minimize the chances of this happening, start the day with a breakfast that includes a complete protein like eggs or cheese on a slice of whole grain bread. Include a fat like coconut oil or avocado to further slow your digestion.

If you don't like eating breakfast then make a smoothie with some almond milk, yogurt, nut butter and a handful of berries. You can drink this while you're doing your morning routine.

There are two schools of thought on structuring the way you eat for the remainder of the day. Some experts claim it is best to eat frequent snacks throughout the day, while others say you should stick to three well balanced meals.

You can choose whichever eating pattern fits your lifestyle. If you have eaten a substantial breakfast, you probably won't feel your energy flagging until lunchtime. If, on the other hand, you drank a smoothie, you may feel your concentration slipping by mid-morning. In this case have a small healthy snack prepared, like a small apple and a piece of cheese or a hardboiled egg.

The points to remember are to include protein, complex carbohydrates, and healthy fats with each meal, or mini-meal. Don't allow yourself to become ravenous. That's when you're likely to become short-tempered, have difficulty concentrating, and this is when you become vulnerable to making bad food choices.

Herbs that can Help Balance Mood

We all go through emotionally challenging times. There's nothing wrong with using an herbal supplement to take the edge off when work is particularly stressful, or if you've suffered a loss and feel like you're not coping well. However, during these times the emotional support you could receive from a good therapist might be more appropriate. A good therapist can help you increase your emotional reserves, develop better coping strategies, and strengthen your current coping mechanisms.

That said, the following list of herbs has been found both safe and effective for short-term use.

Ashwagandha is an adaptogen. Adaptogens appear to have the ability to help regulate homeostasis. They help to balance your mood. In the face of stress one of our physiological responses includes a rise in cortisol. Adaptogens are able to exert an influence over this by targeting the hypothalamic pituitary adrenal axis. They are able to decrease the amount of cortisol and nitric oxide and thereby create a sense of calm. Because it helps restore balance it also reduces fatigue, and helps improve concentration.

Ashwagandha has been used as part of Ayurvedic healing for centuries. Ayurveda is an ancient form of healing practiced in India. There has been a great deal of recent research on this plant. It is generally recognized as safe: however, it is not recommended for use during pregnancy.

Rhodiola is another adaptogen, with a long history of use. This herb has a great deal of recent research supporting its benefits. Like Ashwagandha it is used to improve poor concentration and fatigue. However, where Ashwagandha is used for anxious states, Rhodiola is used in depressed states.

Ginkgo biloba has numerous applications ranging from enhancing brain function to decreasing the effects of cognitive decline in the elderly. One reason why Ginkgo may have a large range of effects on the body may lie in its anti-inflammatory properties. This could be one reason why some of the long-term studies on the elderly have found a decrease in cognitive decline. In a 20-year population-based study on 3,612 people aged 65 or more, researchers found a lower rate of decline in the participants who took Ginkgo biloba extract. (5)

Similarly a review on enhancement of brain function notes that numerous studies have found evidence that Ginkgo biloba taken even in single doses can show an improvement in cognitive function in younger adults. The only cautionary note is to ensure that the extract is standardized due to the toxicity of ginkgolic acid. (46)

Chapter Seven

Mindful eating

Mindful eating is possible when we create the time to become present. This means not eating unconsciously, or when you're distracted. Do you have a morning ritual around breakfast, or do you drink coffee in the car on the way to work? What does lunch look like? Are you able to take a break, or do you eat at your desk? What about dinner? Do you prepare a meal, or do you graze without sitting down?

In the best of all possible worlds, you would be free to enjoy each meal. But realistically most of us simply don't have that luxury. It may take a little practice to learn to recognize your eating patterns. Once you do, you can decide what kind of changes you'd like to make.

I do not like to wake up and eat. However my morning coffee ritual is sacred to me. I make a mug of expresso with homemade nut milk, sprinkled with cinnamon and cocoa. I savor it with no distractions. My dogs curl up with me and we enjoy the quiet together. When I'm finished with it, I feel prepared to start my day centered and focused.

If you're not a morning person, this might not appeal to you. I have a friend who always pours a glass of wine when she begins to cook. That's her signal that the day is over and it's time to relax. So, which meal could become special to you?

Mindfulness and Food Cravings

We all have our vulnerabilities and we are most likely to give in to a craving when we are not prepared for them. It's important to take the time to consider your weekly schedule so you can plan for the nights when you're likely to be rushed, hungry or tired. Our emotions, environments, and situations affect our eating patterns. Some of these days or evenings may be cyclical, for instance feeling exhausted every Friday. Another instance may be when you have had a stressful meeting. If you have children in the house, or a busy evening schedule those could be times when a drive through seems like your best bet for a meal. It's not!

Being prepared gives you more control over your life. You can be proactive not reactive. The difference between the two is huge. Think of a time when you were hungry and tired and you stopped a picked up a burger to eat in the car. Did you enjoy that meal? Did you feel nourished?

Chances are you wolfed it down without even tasting it. This kind of eating can take a toll on your health. If you ate some fries you ingested most likely trans fats, which will have a negative effect on your cholesterol. The meal would have been high in sodium impacting your blood pressure and coronary health. It would also have been high in simple carbohydrates, which if not burned will be stored as fat.

Now consider another scenario. On Saturday you looked at your schedule for the week and noted two evenings when you would be very busy. You considered a couple of options for healthy meals that you could pull out the refrigerator and eat before leaving for the next event. You prepared this meal along with your lunch the evening before so you would not be rushed.

In the above scenario, the situation that led to poor eating was a time constraint. Other situations can include eating meals alone, snacking at your desk, or eating in front of the TV. The emotions involved were hunger and fatigue. Other feelings can include boredom, loneliness, sorrow, or anxiety. In the above scenario the situational trigger is a time constraint. What would some healthy coping strategies look like?

Practicing good self-care when you feel, lonely, sad, anxious...try taking a bath, lighting a candle, taking a walk, painting your nails, take up a new hobby, try knitting, join a yoga class, what about belly dancing, get a library card and visit the library, take a cooking class. The options are endless. Just remember; If you always do what you always did, you'll always get what you always got.

Mindfulness and Our Senses

Being mindful can also help us to recognize our eating cues. Do you eat according to the clock, in response to the sight or smell of food, or when you feel hungry? Sometimes when we eat is a matter of practicality, like you get your lunch break at noon. Other times we may find that we're so engrossed in a project that we don't even notice that we're hungry. However, our senses can override both of these scenarios.

We rely on all of our senses as we go through each day. Listening, smelling, touching and watching. Eating is very much a sensory experience. Each of our senses heightens the experience when we have a meal.

The Eyes

There is a saying that we eat with our eyes. Use of color is visually enticing. Consider the options below:

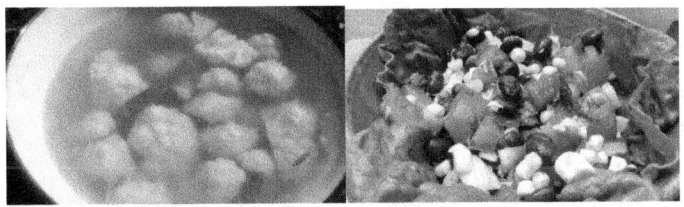

Marketers are well aware of this. Have you ever become hungry while watching a cooking show, or when reading a recipe in a magazine? This is because we become stimulated upon seeing food. We expect that based on its appearance it would taste good.

The Nose

The sense of smell is a vital part of the eating experience. Without smell we are still able to discern some of the flavors, such as sweet or bitter, but the aroma is lost. The sense of smell alerts us to danger (think smoke), as well as rewards. Scents are associated with people, places and things.

Our sense of smell is highly attuned. We are able to discern thousands of different scents. We are also quick to notice the smell of favorite foods. Once the smell of food has been detected, our bodies begin to prepare for a meal. The mouth begins to water, digestive juices start to flow and hunger intensifies.

The Mouth

Flavor is detected on our tongues. We can identify five distinct flavors. They are:

Salty, abundant in sea vegetables and found in fish

Savory, usually found in meats and animal products, also seaweed

Sweet, occurs naturally in fruit and some vegetables

Sour, can also be found in fruit

Bitter, is found in vegetables and seeds

Astringency and pungency are sensations, not flavors. Astringency is perceived when tannins from wine or tea touch the tongue. Pungency refers to the sensations from a hot vegetable like peppers, ginger or horseradish.

Incorporating Fat, Acid, Salt and Sweet (FASS) to Improve Taste

There are four factors that affect our perception of taste. When we cook, we aspire to achieve balance between these:

Fat: This adds texture to the dish and rounds out the other flavors

Acid: This is the first flavor perceived in a dish, it is a high note

Salt: This enhances the flavor of a dish and balances acid and sweet

Sweet: This lingers on the palate and balances salt and acid, it is a low note

Aroma and the sense of Smell

Smell is a huge part of the eating experience, even more so than our eyes, which prepare us for a meal. The sense of smell is seated in the most primal part of the brain. It is linked to the centers for memory, emotion and language in the basal ganglia. It is closely linked to the centers for memory, emotion and language. This proximity is the reason we can be transported back to earlier memories so easily when we smell certain foods.

These are some of the aromas we can detect:

Green, found in green vegetables and some apple skins

Fruity, found in fruits, most notable in stronger fruits and as fruits ripen

Earthy, found in mushroom, beets and in some yeasty breads

Floral, found in fermented fruits, honey and edible flowers like lavender

Spicy, often refers to cinnamon, allspice and nutmeg, but can be hot too

Citrus, citrus fruits like lemon, limes, oranges, grapefruit

Sulphur, refers to onions, garlic and hard boiled eggs

Nutty, generally refers to nuts but can also refer to caramel or molasses

Taste and Texture, and Temperature

Texture is the part of the eating experience in which your mouth uses sensation, much the way your hands use the sense of touch. Consider velvet or sharp as both a taste sensation and something to touch. They are perceived in similar ways.

Temperature affects the flavor. As a food is warmed the flavors become stronger. This is particularly true of salty foods. Salt is perceived as stronger when the food is cold.

Consistency affects the flavor of food. Thicker foods are usually perceived as having a milder taste.

Mouthfeel is the combination of smell, texture, temperature, and taste.

The Environment

A final component to a perfect meal is the ambience. Memorable meals are based on much more than just the food. The atmosphere of the environment is a big part as well.

The difference between feeling relaxed and welcome versus feeling overwhelmed and stressed can be felt as soon as you enter a space. A cluttered or chaotic environment creates a very different experience than one that is neat and organized.

In one setting we could be offered a gourmet meal and not fully enjoy it because of the distractions. In the peaceful environment we could just eat cheese and be very happy with it.

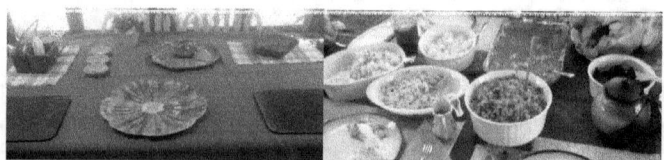

These two setting are in the same room at my house. In one instance I was rushed and much more focused on getting the food on the table, so much so that you can't even see the place settings. In the other picture the food is not yet on the table, but I was very focused on creating a peaceful ambience. You'll have to take my word that once the food was on the table it did not appear cluttered.

Here is a general rule of thumb to keep in mind when setting the table. This includes planning for a party, or a party of one:

Peaceful: clean table, dimmable lighting, candles, flowers, soft music all lead to a relaxing evening.

Problematic: clutter, bright lights, few or no decorations do not create a calming and welcoming environment.

If you're hosting a party, plan to have food in more than one location. Snacks like nuts can go in on an end table along with a stack of small napkins. Beverages should be set up in another location with glasses/cups and ice. Desserts should be in a cooler area along with small plates, napkins, and forks. The main course can either remain in the kitchen or be served on the table depending on the type of party, and number of guests.

These pointers can help you feel more relaxed and help your guests feel more welcome.

Part Four

Chapter Eight

Specialized Diets

Three diets that people have had a great deal of success in using to help decrease digestive disorders are the Low- FODMAP Diet, the Gut and Psychology Syndrome Diet (the GAPS Diet) and the Specific Carbohydrate Diet (SCD). These are complicated diets that follow specific protocols. There are long lists of foods that are allowed and foods that are prohibited. Each of these diets have books, websites, and blogs to support anyone who wishes to utilize them. They are well-researched and have helped many people.

In familiarizing myself with these diets I noticed that there are a few foods that are allowed on all of the diets and a few foods that are prohibited on each of these diets. It may be worthwhile to limit yourself to the foods that everyone can eat to see if this helps you. If it does you can do more research to see which diet will work for you long-term.

Foods allowed on SCD, GAPS, and FODMAP

Meats: Fresh or frozen, not processed, chicken, turkey, beef, pork, lamb

Fish and Seafood, fresh or frozen, not processed, or smoked

Vegetables: Broccoli, brussel sprouts, cabbage, carrots, celery (in small amounts), cucumbers, kale, lettuce, pumpkin, spinach, squash, string beans, tomatoes

Fruit: Bananas (ripe with black spots), berries, coconut, grapes, kiwi, lemons, limes, melons, oranges, pineapples

Dairy: Eggs, butter, dry curd cottage cheese (aka Farmers cheese)

Nuts: Almonds, brazil nuts, hazel nuts, pecans, walnuts

Legumes: Lentils

Foods not allowed on any of the diets

Cereal and Grain: Wheat, barley, rye, rice, spelt

Processed meats

Soybeans

Milk

Elimination diet

Elimination diets are recommended for many reasons. These include treating inflammation and digestive disorders, and uncovering food sensitivities. It is one of the first things I recommend when someone tells me they are suffering from headaches, aching joints, stuffy sinuses or congested ears, digestive disturbances, or skin problems.

When doing an elimination diet, it should be followed for at least one month. The foods that should be eliminated include:

Sugar

Wheat

Corn

Dairy

Soy

Processed food

When people hear that they need to remove these foods from their diets they almost always say, "Well what does that leave?" My answer is everything else.

After you have lived without these potential triggers for at least two weeks, though a month is better, you will reintroduce one type of food at a time. So using wheat as an example, at the end of the elimination diet period, you would have a wheat based cereal for breakfast, a sandwich for lunch and pasta for dinner. Then wait to see how you feel the next day. If you find your symptoms returning, remove that food again and try it again in one month. Wait at least two days before reintroducing another food and follow the same pattern, e.g., milk for breakfast, yogurt for lunch and something in a cream sauce for dinner.

If the lining of your digestive tract is very badly damaged it may take up to six months to heal. At that time you may be able to tolerate small amounts of foods that may have been triggers, though you may find instead there are foods you may have to live without in order to feel well.

Foods that should not be reintroduced are processed foods, foods high in sugar, and foods high in saturated fat.

Gluten-Free

Gluten-free diets have been adopted by many people. Some people are following what they think is a healthier way of eating. For other people it is truly a serious health issue. People with Celiac disease cannot ever have any wheat, period. People with wheat sensitivities may be able to occasionally have a little wheat, but they will most likely suffer a range of symptoms including digestive disturbances.

The abundance of gluten-free products on the market is both confusing and overwhelming. Because of the confusion, savvy marketers have jumped on the gluten-free bandwagon. These products are no healthier than the originals. They have preservatives, too much salt, too much sugar, and unhealthy fats.

It is important to read the labels of anything that is gluten-free. Oats are gluten-free, but they should come from a mill that does not process wheat.

Another substitute for wheat flour includes beans. Beans can be used in a cooked form, or dried and ground as a flour. I use chick peas and black beans in several of my recipes. I prefer them cooked to dry because the ground flours tend to be bitter.

I like to use a short-cut for my baking needs. This standard mix can be used for making everything from pancakes and apple fritters to pies and cookies. It can also be modified according to your specific dietary needs and personal taste.

½ cup oat flour
¼ cup sorghum flour
¼ cup coconut, rice flour or almond flour
¼ tapioca flour or potato starch

This can be used in place of wheat flour.

Here's an easy cookie recipe:

1 ¼ cup of above flour mix
¾ cup butter or coconut oil
1 egg
¼ cup agave
1 tsp. vanilla
1 tsp. baking soda
½ tsp salt

Blend the butter, egg, vanilla and agave until smooth. Add baking soda and salt to the flour and slowly add to the butter mixture. This will be a very soft batter. It can be used in a cookie press or be rolled into logs, refrigerated then sliced into cookies. In either case bake in an oved pre-heated to 325° for 8-10 minutes. Cool and eat as-is or top with melted chocolate.

Raw Food

People usually go on raw food diets as a detoxification strategy. It is important to remember the basic components of good nutrition. Protein, carbohydrates, and healthy fats are all part of a well-balanced diet. This type of diet tends to be low in protein, so if you choose to follow this type of eating plan be sure to add raw nuts and beans to your meals.

Alternatively, you could consider following a mostly raw diet and incorporate some cooked meat and fish. A healthy person should have no problem having juices and raw food as the base of their diet. You could also follow a seasonal diet, that's my preference.

When spring green begin to come up, start substituting them for heavier root vegetables that are available during autumn and winter. As more spring and summer fruits and vegetables become available keep adding them to your diet.

A nice smoothie or juice for breakfast, raw soup for lunch, and salad for dinner is a healthy way to eat when your body needs hydration. If you find you're rushed in the morning, juice can be made the night before it will be used. It will lose many of its enzymes after 24 hours, so don't make a large batch and plan to drink it all week long.

When preparing raw meals try to use 3 vegetables to each fruit. Many people make smoothies that are all fruit. An excess of fruit provides too much sugar at one time, so don't forget the veggies!

I love making raw soups during the warm months. This is a basic recipe that can be modified using different herbs or vegetables.

Raw Cucumber Soup

2 cucumbers

1 clove garlic

½ an onion

1 tsp. dill

1 tsp. salt

1 Tbs. coconut vinegar

1 Tbs. cold-pressed olive oil

Blend all ingredients in food processor until chunky.

Vegan Diet

The difference between a vegan and a vegetarian can be most easily illustrated below:

Semi Vegetarians eat chicken

Pescatarians eat fish

Lacto-vegetarians eat dairy

Ovo-vegetarians eat eggs

Vegans eat none of the above

Vegans are also sometimes called "strict" vegetarians. They simply don't eat animal products. Many follow this eating pattern for ethical reasons, some for health reasons, and some for religious reasons. Whatever the case, they are not as difficult to feed as people think they might be.

There are numerous food options available. Explore different ethnic foods such as Indian, Chinese, Mexican, and Asian. These all have many vegetarian and vegan recipes.

The easiest way to look at having a vegan over for dinner is to once again consider what the body needs, protein, fat and carbohydrate. People who are not used to cooking for a vegan become the most overwhelmed by protein sources. Plant sources include quinoa, soy, seeds, beans, pulses, and nuts.

An easy meal to feed a vegan starts with a grain base. Add some vegetables to that and finish it with a plant protein.

Tabbouleh

2 Tbs. chopped scallions

4 large tomatoes, chopped

1 large cucumber, chopped

½ cup chick peas

3 lemons, (Freshly Squeezed)

5 tablespoons olive oil

1 cup bulgur

1 cup water, boiled

1 cup parsley, minced

1/8 teaspoon ground black pepper

1/4 teaspoon salt

Add one cup of boiled water and one cup of bulgur in a small bowl and mix. Place a towel over the bowl so the steam is unable to escape. Set aside until cool. Add remaining ingredients.

Diet Trends

Diet trends are as old as human kind. Human beings are naturally inquisitive. When we hear, or read about something new we want to try it ourselves. I'm no exception to this. I would guess over 50 cook books line a few of my shelves and easily another 50 books on specific diets line additional shelves.

Diet trends like macrobiotic cooking, Mediterranean and Paleolithic (paleo) diets can be healthy alternatives for someone interested in changing the way they eat. Diets like master cleanse, the cabbage soup diet, or the grape fruit diet, are not going to meet our nutritional needs.

For the past few decades the guiding principle has been to follow a low fat diet. This was followed by the low carbohydrate diets. Now the trend is heading toward a high fat diet.

Diet aside, we lead increasingly sedentary lifestyles. Someone asked me recently, upon seeing the size of my lawn what kind of tractor I had. I said I'm the tractor. Seriously, I may not be a big fan of mowing the lawn, but I welcome the exercise.

In the end this is what it boils down to, eat a balanced whole food diet, exercise every day, sleep 7 to 8 hours every night, spend time in social settings, and relax or meditate.

Hypocrites said "Let food be thy medicine" over 2,000 years ago. Food is foundational to our well-being. However, calories in calories out is a bit too simplistic. Leading a balanced life is the key to better health.

Acknowledgements

This book is dedicated to my mother and grandmother because they were my first teachers. Nutrition was a regular point of discussion and we paid attention.

Maryland University of Integrative Health had the wisdom to bring extremely talented chefs to the school to teach the nutrition students the art of creating food as medicine. Among them Chef Jill Gusman, and Chef Myra Kornfeld were the most inspiring. All the visiting chefs were supervised by Chef Eleonora Grafton. Her knowledge and humor enriched the cooking labs.

While attending MUIH I had the opportunity meet some wonderful women who made a big impact on me. Jen Swartout, who opened her home to me while I was attending the week-long classes so many miles from my home. Jen Brennan my walking buddy. Yevgeniya Libkhen my sometimes cooking partner, who wrote a letter of recommendation in order that I could sit for the CNS exam.

I worked in groups with several fellow students on intensive research projects. The section on migraines and Lyme disease was based on our work. They were Jennifer Brennan, Jennifer Swartout, Andrea Strohecker, Courtney Struthers, Traci McKenzie-Knight, Jamie Abbaticchio, and Jason Bosley-Smith.

I want to acknowledge my friends who supported of my radical idea to return to school. The first is Alice Forsyth who was my guiding light. The second is Liz Ryan, the writer of Reinvention Roadmap. The third is Angie Helms who moved to Grand Caymen, and invited us to visit. This is where all our ideas were born.

This book would not have been finished without the assistance of my brother Phillip. He kindly read my first draft and told me what areas needed more work.

This book would not have been published without the keen editorial eye of my husband Bob, who spent hours correcting my drafts.

Nothing in my life would be possible without the love of my children Elizabeth and David and my precious grandson Robbie (and his mommy Loni).

References

1. Abdallah Ismail, N., Ragab, S. H., Abd ElBaky, A., Shoeib, A. R. S., Alhosary, Y., & Fekry, D. (2011). Frequency of Firmicutes and Bacteroidetes in gut microbiota in obese and normal weight Egyptian children and adults. Archives of Medical Science : AMS, 7(3), 501–507.
2. Altman, R. (2010). Early Management of Osteoarthritis. American Journal Of Managed Care, 16S41-S47.
3. Amen, D.G. Change Your Brain Change Your Body, 2010, New York, NY: Three Rivers Press.
4. Amen, D.G. Change Your Brain Change Your Life, 1998, New York, NY: Three Rivers Press.
5. Amieva, H., Meillon, C., Helmer, C., Barberger-Gateau, P., &Dartigues, J. (2013). Ginkgo Biloba Extract and Long-Term Cognitive Decline: A 20-Year Follow-Up Population-Based Study. Plos ONE, 8(1), 1-8. doi:10.1371/journal.pone.0052755
6. Asemi, Z., Samimi, M., Tabassi, Z., Sabihi, S., &Esmaillzadeh, A. (2013). A randomized controlled clinical trial investigating the effect of DASH diet on insulin resistance, inflammation, and oxidative stress in gestational diabetes. Nutrition, 29(4), 619-624. doi:10.1016/j.nut.2012.11.020
7. Baigent, C. (2013). Vascular and upper gastrointestinal effects of non-steroidal anti-inflammatory drugs: meta-analyses of individual participant data from randomised trials. Lancet, 382(9894), 769-779. doi:10.10161S0140-6736(13)60900-9
8. Balch, P. and Balch, J. (2000). Prescription for Nutritional Healing. 3e, New York, NY: Penguin Putnam Inc.
9. Blum, S. (2013). The Immune System Recovery Plan, New York, NY: Scribner.
10. Bilal Ahmad, Muneeb U. Rehman, Insha Amin, et al., "A Review on Pharmacological Properties of Zingerone (4-(4-Hydroxy-3-methoxyphenyl)-2-butanone)," The Scientific World Journal, vol. 2015, Article ID 816364, 6 pages, 2015. doi:10.1155/2015/816364
11. Bone, K. & Mills, S. (2012). Principles and Practice of Phytotherapy, 2nd ed.: Modern herbal medicine. Australia: Churchill LivingstoneWeiss.
12. Bozic, K., Bashyal, R., Anthony, S., Chiu, V., Shulman, B., &Rubash, H. (2013). Is Administratively Coded Comorbidity and Complication Data in Total Joint Arthroplasty Valid?. Clinical Orthopaedics& Related Research, 471(1), 201-205. doi:10.1007/s11999-012-2352-1
13. Braun, L., and Cohen, M. (2010). Herbs and Natural Supplements, an Evidence-based Guide, 3e, Oxford, Elsevier Health Sciences.
14. Buhner, S. (2012). Herbal Antibiotics, Natural Alternatives for Treating Drug-Resistant Bacteria, 2e, North Adams, MA: Storey Publishing.
15. Bures, J, Cyrany,J, Kohoutova, D, Förstl, M, Rejchrt S, Kvetina, J, Vorisek, V, Kopacova, M. Small intestinal bacterial overgrowth syndrome. World J Gastroenterol (2010). 16(24): 2978-2990
16. Bye W, Ishaq N, Bolin TD, Duncombe VM, Riordan SM. Overgrowth of the indigenous gut microbiome and irritable bowel syndrome. World J Gastroenterol (2014). 20(10): 2449-2455.
17. Campbell, Y., Fantacone, M., &Gombart, A. (2012). Regulation of antimicrobial peptide gene expression by nutrients and by-products of microbial metabolism. European Journal Of Nutrition, 51(8), 899-907. doi:10.1007/s00394-012-0415-4.

18. Campbell-McBride, N. (2010). Gut and Psychology Syndrome, United Kingdom: Medinform Publishing.
19. Carvalho, B., &Saad, M. (2013). Influence of gut microbiota on subclinical inflammation and insulin resistance. Mediators Of Inflammation, 2013986734. doi:10.1155/2013/986734.
20. Chan, F., Cryer, B., Goldstein, J., Lanas, A., Peura, D., Scheiman, J., & ... Dodge, W. (2010). A novel composite endpoint to evaluate the gastrointestinal (GI) effects of nonsteroidal antiinflammatory drugs through the entire GI tract. Journal Of Rheumatology, 37(1), 167-174. doi:10.3899/jrheum.090168.
21. Chatterjee, P. et. al. (2012). Evaluation of anti-inflammatory effects of green tea and black tea: A comparative in vitro study. J Adv Pharm Technol Res. 2012 Apr-Jun; 3(2): 136–138. doi: 10.4103/2231-4040.97298 PMCID: PMC3401676.
22. Chedid V. et. al. (2014). Herbal therapy is equivalent to rifaximin for the treatment of small intestinal bacterial overgrowth. Glob Adv Health Med. 2014 May;3(3):16-24. doi: 10.7453/gahmj.2014.019.
23. Colbin, A. (1986). Food and Healing, New York, NY: Ballantine Books.
24. Delzenne, N. M., Neyrinck, A. M., &Cani, P. D. (2011). Modulation of the gut microbiota by nutrients with prebiotic properties: consequences for host health in the context of obesity and metabolic syndrome. Microbial Cell Factories, 10(Suppl 1), 1-11. doi:10.1186/1475-2859-10-S1-S10.
25. DesMiisons, K. (1998). Potatoes Not Prozac, New York, NY: Simon & Schuster.
26. Duke, J. (1997). The Green Pharmacy. New York, NY: Rodale Press.
27. Estruch, R. et al. (2013). Primary Prevention of Cardiovascular Disease with a Mediterranean Diet. N Engl J Med 2013; 368:1279-1290April 4, 2013DOI: 10.1056/NEJMoa1200303
28. Fallon, S. (2001). Nourishing Traditions. 2nd E. Washington, DC: New Trends Publishing Inc.
29. Forsythe, P., Kunze, W., &Bienenstock, J. (2012). On communication between gut microbes and the brain. Current Opinion In Gastroenterology, 28(6), 557-562. doi:10.1097/MOG.0b013e3283572ffa.
30. Gottschall, E. (1986). Breaking the Vicious Cycle, Canada: Kirkton Press.
31. Henrotin, Y., Priem, F., &Mobasheri, A. (2013). Curcumin: a new paradigm and therapeutic opportunity for the treatment of osteoarthritis: curcumin for osteoarthritis management. Springerplus, 2(1), 56.
32. Huff, E. People Who Eat Processed Junk Food are Angry, Irritable, say Scientists. http://www.naturalnews.com/039655_processed_food_irritability_research.html
33. Hyman, M. (2005). Ultraprevention, New York, NY: Atria Books.
34. Jennings, A., Welch, A., Fairweather-Tait, S., Kay, C., Minihane, A., Chowienczyk, P., & ... Cassidy, A. (2012). Higher anthocyanin intake is associated with lower arterial stiffness and central blood pressure in women. The American Journal Of Clinical Nutrition, 96(4), 781-788.
35. Katiyar, S., & Raman, C. (2011). Green tea: a new option for the prevention or control of osteoarthritis. Arthritis Research & Therapy, 13(4), 121. doi:10.1186/ar3428.

36. Kau, A., et. al. Human nutrition, the gut microbiome, and immune system: envisioning the future. Nature. 2011 Jun 15; 474(7351): 327–336.

37. Kennedy, D., & Wightman, E. (2011). Herbal extracts and phytochemicals: plant secondary metabolites and the enhancement of human brain function. Advances In Nutrition (Bethesda, Md.), 2(1), 32-50. doi:10.3945/an.110.000117.

38. Klein-Wieringa, I., Kloppenburg, M., Bastiaansen-Jenniskens, Y., Yusuf, E., Kwekkeboom, J., El-Bannoudi, H., & ... Ioan-Facsinay, A. (2011). The infrapatellar fat pad of patients with osteoarthritis has an inflammatory phenotype. Annals Of The Rheumatic Diseases, 70(5), 851-857. doi:10.1136/ard.2010.140046.

39. Lindseth G., Coolahan SE, Petros TV, Lindseth PD.Neurobehavioral Effects of Aspartame Consumption.Res Nurs Health. 2014 Jun; 37(3):185-93. doi: 10.1002/nur.21595. Epub 2014 Apr 3.

40. Lipski, E. (2012). Digestive Wellness, 4th ed.: Strengthen the Immune System and Prevent Disease Through Healthy Digestion. New York, McGraw Hill.

41. Lopez, H. (2012). Nutritional interventions to prevent and treat osteoarthritis. Part II: focus on micronutrients and supportive nutraceuticals. PM & R: The Journal Of Injury, Function, And Rehabilitation, 4(5 Suppl), S155-S168. doi:10.1016/j.pmrj.2012.02.023.

42. Luckey, D., Gomez, A., Murray, J., White, B., &Taneja, V. (2013). Bugs & us: The role of the gut in autoimmunity. Indian Journal of Medical Research, 138(5), 732-743.

43. Mayer, E. (2016). The Mind-Gut Connection, New York, NY: HarperCollins Books.

44. McGee, H.(2004). On Food and Cooking, New York, NY: Scribner.

45. Meyers, A. (2016). The Thyroid Connection, New York, NY: Little, Brown and Company.

46. Morais, C. et.al. (2016). Anthocyanins as inflammatory modulators and the role of the gut microbiota. The Journal of Nutritional Biochemistry, Volume 33, July 2016, Pages 1–7.

47. Ou, H., Hsieh, Y., Yang, N., Tsai, K., Chen, K., Tsai, C., & ... Lee, S. (2013). Ginkgo biloba extract attenuates oxLDL-induced endothelial dysfunction via an AMPK-dependent mechanism. Journal Of Applied Physiology (Bethesda, Md.: 1985), 114(2), 274-285. doi:10.1152/japplphysiol.00367.2012.

48. Pandey, K.B. and Rizvi, S.I. Plant polyphenols as dietary antioxidants in human health and disease. Oxid Med Cell Longev. 2009 Nov-Dec; 2(5): 270–278. doi: 10.4161/oxim.2.5.9498 PMCID: PMC2835915.

49. Parkinson, L. and Keast, R. (2014). Oleocanthal, a Phenolic Derived from Virgin Olive Oil: A Review of the Beneficial Effects on Inflammatory Disease. Int J Mol Sci. 2014 Jul; 15(7): 12323–12334. Published online 2014 Jul 11. doi: 10.3390/ijms150712323. PMCID: PMC4139846.

50. Perlmutter, D. (2015). Brain Maker, New York, NY: Little, Brown and Company.

51. Petrucci, K. (2015). Dr. Kellyann's Bone Broth Diet. New York, NY: Rodale Inc.

52. Pottenger, F. (1983). Pottenger's Cats, a Study in Nutrition, Lemon Grove CA: Price-Pottenger Nutrition Foundation.

53. Provino, R. (2010). The role of adaptogens in stress management. Australian Journal Of Medical Herbalism, 22(2), 41-49.

54. Reinisalo, Et. Al. Polyphenol Stilbenes: Molecular Mechanisms of Defence against Oxidative Stress and Aging-Related Diseases. Oxidative Medicine and Cellular Longevity, Volume 2015 (2015), Article ID 340520, 24 pages http://dx.doi.org/10.1155/2015/340520.

55. Sabater-Molina, Larqué E, Torrella F, Zamora S.J PhysiolBiochem. 2009. Dietary fructooligosaccharides and potential benefits on health.Sep;65(3):315-28. doi: 10.1007/BF03180584.

56. Sanders, M., &Grundmann, O. (2011). The Use of Glucosamine, Devil's Claw (Harpagophytumprocumbens), and Acupuncture as Complementary and Alternative Treatments for Osteoarthritis. Alternative Medicine Review, 16(3), 228-238.

57. Shealy, C. (2002). Healing Remedies. London: Harper Collins Publishers.

58. Shepherd, S. and Gibson, P. (2013). The Low FODMAP Diet, New York, NY: The Experiment, LLC.

59. Simmons, D. (2008). Epigenetic influence and disease. Nature Education 1(1):6.

60. Skenderi, G. (2003). Herbal vade mecum. Rutherford, NJ: Herbacy Press.

61. Stilling, R. M., Dinan, T. G., & Cryan, J. F. (2014). Microbial genes, brain & behaviour - epigenetic regulation of the gut-brain axis. Genes, Brain & Behavior, 13(1), 69-86. doi:10.1111/gbb.12109.

62. Stipanuk, M. Caudill, M. (2013). Biochemical, Physiological, and Molecular Aspects of Human Nutrition, 3rd ed. St. Louis, MO: Elsevier Saunders.

63. Stoler, D. Transfats Bad for Your Brain, 2015, https://www.psychologytoday.com/blog/the-resilient-brain/201506/trans-fats-bad-your-brain.

64. Swain, M. R., Anandharaj, M., Ray, R. C., & Parveen Rani, R. (2014). Fermented Fruits and Vegetables of Asia: A Potential Source of Probiotics. Biotechnology Research International, 2014, 250424. http://doi.org/10.1155/2014/250424.

65. Tillisch, K., Labus, J., Kilpatrick, L., Jiang, Z., Stains, J., Ebrat, B., & ... Mayer, E. (2013). Consumption of fermented milk product with probiotic modulates brain activity. Gastroenterology, 144(7), 1394. doi:10.1053/j.gastro.2013.02.043.

66. Tomé-Carneiro, M. Gonzálvez, M. Larrosa et al., "Grape resveratrol increases serum adiponectin and downregulates inflammatory genes in peripheral blood mononuclear cells: a triple-blind, placebo-controlled, one-year clinical trial in patients with stable coronary artery disease," Cardiovascular Drugs and Therapy, vol. 27, no. 1, pp. 37–48, 2013.

67. Valussi, M. (2012). Functional foods with digestion-enhancing properties. International Journal Of Food Sciences & Nutrition, 6382-89. doi:10.3109/09637486.2011.627841

68. Vanharanta M, Voutilainen S, Rissanen TH, Adlercreutz H, Salonen JT. Risk of cardiovascular disease-related and all-cause death according to serum concentrations of enterolactone: Kuopio Ischaemic Heart Disease Risk Factor Study. Arch Intern Med. 2003; 163(9):1099-1104.

69. Vegezzi G, Anselmi L, Huynh J, Barocelli E, Rozengurt E, Raybould H, et al. (2014) Diet-Induced Regulation of Bitter Taste Receptor Subtypes in the Mouse Gastrointestinal Tract. PLoS ONE 9(9): e107732. https://doi.org/10.1371/journal.pone.0107732

70. Yoon, J., &Baek, S. (2005). Molecular targets of dietary polyphenols with anti-inflammatory properties. Yonsei Medical Journal, 46(5), 585-596.

71. Zhang, J.M. and An, J. Cytokines, Inflammation and Pain (2007). Int Anesthesiol Clin. 2007 Spring; 45(2): 27–37. doi: 10.1097/AIA.0b013e318034194e.

72. Zintzaras, E., Kitsios, G. D., Ziogas, D. C., Rodopoulou, P., &Karachalios, T. (2010). Field Synopsis and Synthesis of Genetic Association Studies in Osteoarthritis: The CUMAGAS-OSTEO Information System. American Journal Of Epidemiology, 171(8), 851-858. doi:10.1093/aje/kwq016

73. Omega-3 fatty acids, Maryland University Medical Center, http://umm.edu/health/medical/altmed/supplement/omega3-fatty-acids.

74. Quercetin, Maryland University Medical Center, http://umm.edu/health/medical/altmed/supplement/quercetin.

75. Tyrosine, University of Maryland Medical Center, http://umm.edu/health/medical/altmed/supplement/tyrosine.

76. The Secrets of Resveratrol's Health Benefitshttp://articles.mercola.com/sites/articles/archive/2009/08/18/the-secrets-of-resveratrols-health-benefits.aspx.

77. Lignans, Oregon State University, http://lpi.oregonstate.edu/mic/dietary-factors/phytochemicals/lignans.

www.ingramcontent.com/pod-product-compliance
Lightning Source LLC
Chambersburg PA
CBHW062054280526
45788CB00003B/1218